Deliciously Holistic
Inspired Favorites

VALERIE PENZ

Shellback Publishing, LLC

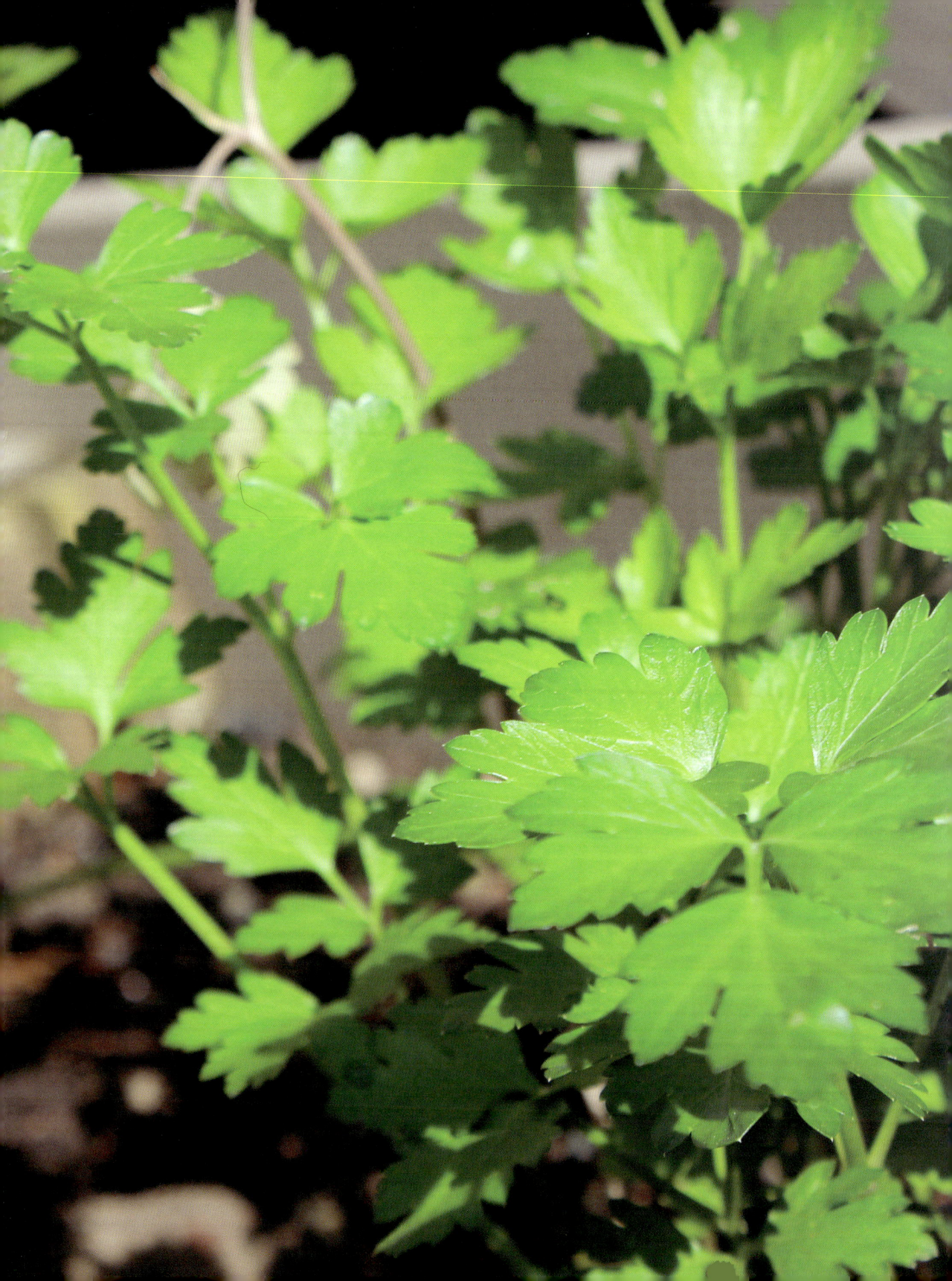

Deliciously Holistic

Inspired Favorites

VALERIE PENZ

Certified Nutritional Therapist and Wellness Coach
Founder of Holistic Health by Valerie

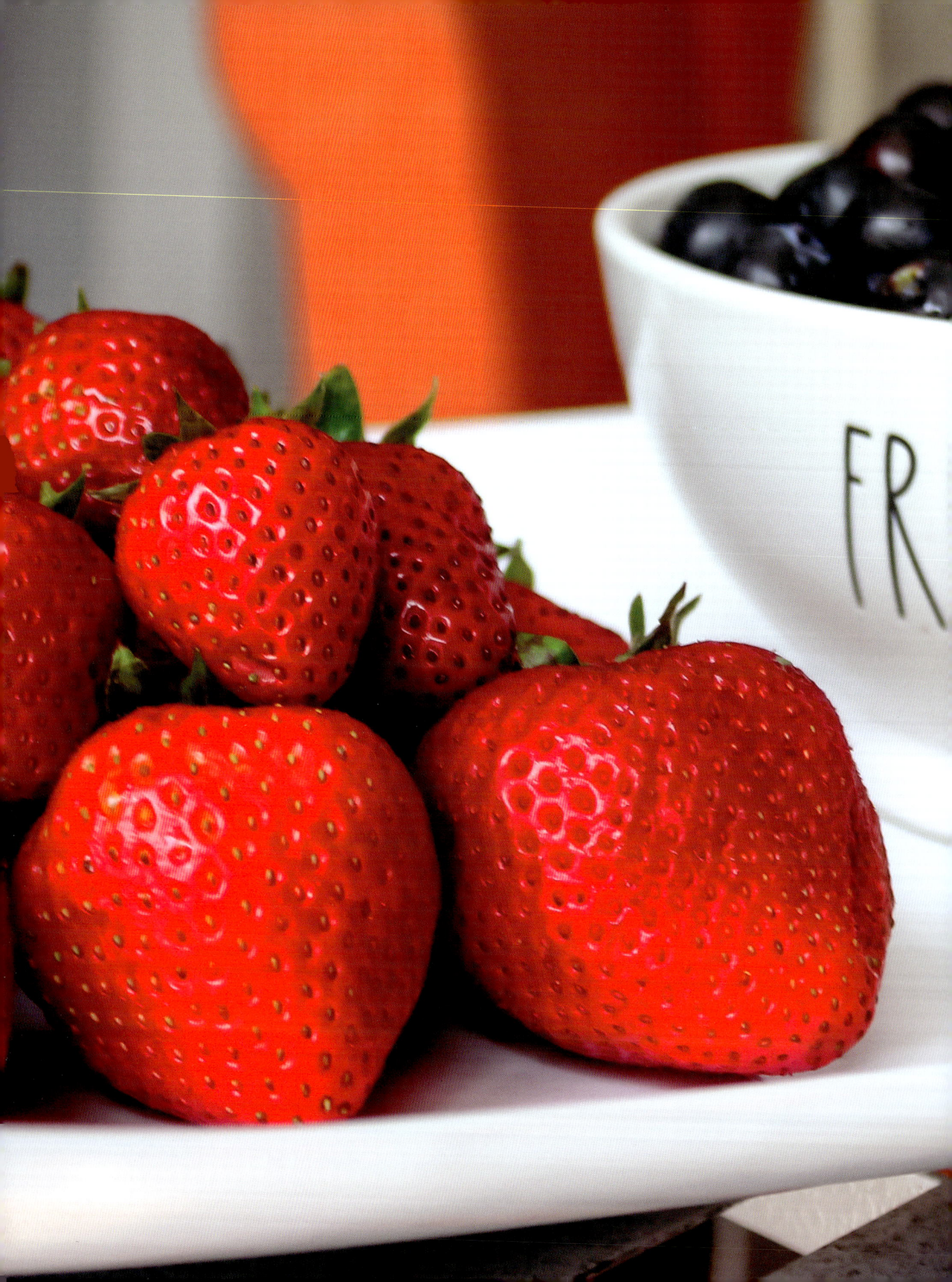

"This cookbook explores how to make enticing, interesting meals that are packed with nutrients without being complicated, expensive, or filled with dairy, gluten, corn, or refined sugars. With over 5 dozen recipes, the author offers a variety to choose from, with every recipe including a short snippet from the author about the recipe's history, practicality, or purpose."

FROM THE BOOK REVIEW DIRECTORY
WWW.BOOKREVIEWDIRECTORY.COM

"I can see this cookbook being one I reach for again and again. There are so many recipes that I can't wait to try. If you are a cookbook lover, and you like to cook healthy, wonderful tasting dishes that are sure to please even the pickiest of eaters then yours truly recommends you add Deliciously Holistic to your collection ASAP."

FROM BETWEEN THE BOOKENDS
WWW.BETWEENTHEBOOKENDS.RECINELLA.DK

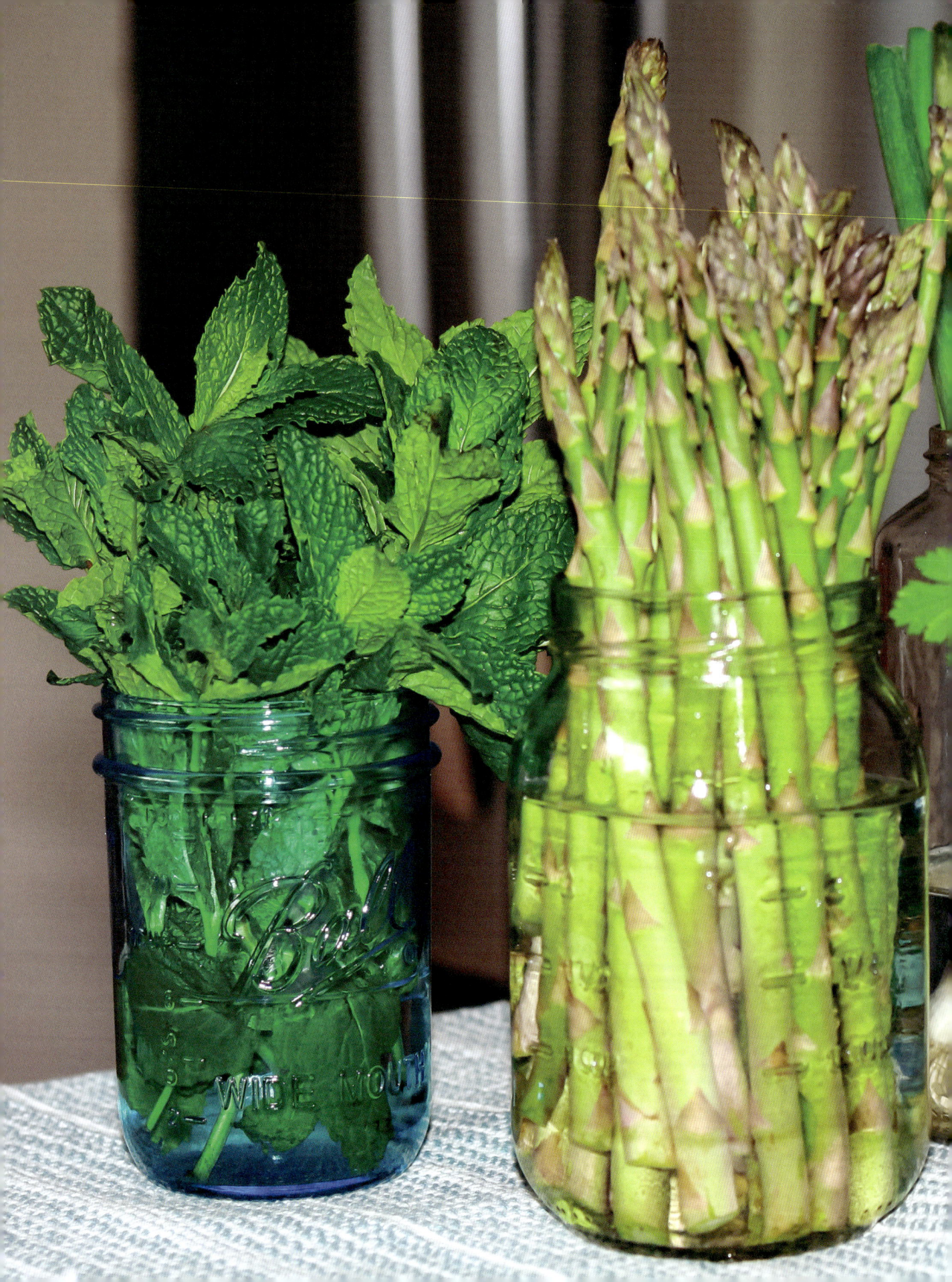

"Deliciously Holistic—Inspired Favorites is written by a nutritional therapist who debunks the myths that eating well involves expense, time, or the need to consume unappetizing fare for the sake of healthy eating.

There are many healthy, natural, holistic cookbooks on the market these days; but Deliciously Holistic—Inspired Favorites stands out from most with its tested, flavor-filled dishes, mouth-watering color photos of completed dishes, ease of preparation, and an approach that combines healthier eating goals with flavors that can't be beat.

Anyone looking to make the transition into better eating should start with Deliciously Holistic—Inspired Favorites. It's a foolproof way of engaging cook and diner over a delicious culinary experience."

FROM THE MIDWEST BOOK REVIEW
WWW.MIDWESTBOOKREVIEW.COM

"I am continually on the lookout for foods that not only taste good, but are made from real food and not hard to make. Valerie Penz provides exactly that. These recipes are ridiculously delicious, affordable, easy to make, and are good for you too!"

FROM NOW DEB
WWW.NOWDEB.COM

Published by Shellback Publishing, LLC

Copyright 2019 by Valerie Penz

All rights reserved. No part of this book may be copied, reproduced or redistributed in any form without the prior written consent of Valerie Penz and Shellback Publishing, LLC.

Disclaimer: This book is intended to supplement an active and healthy lifestyle and does not replace the advice from a medical professional. If you know or suspect you may have a potential or chronic physical or emotional condition, you should contact a medical professional immediately. Shellback Publishing, LLC, Holistic Health by Valerie, LLC and Valerie Penz shall have neither liability nor responsibility for any consequence, directly or indirectly, as a result of the use or application of the contents in this book.

1st printing 2019
ISBN: 978-1-7333358-0-5 (paperback)
ISBN: 978-1-7333358-1-2 (E-Book)
Library of Congress Control Number: 2019913148

Shellback Publishing, LLC
P.O. Box 323, Lake Orion MI 48361
248-834-3059
Shellbackpublishing@gmail.com
Deliciously Holistic—Inspired Favorites

Cover and book layout design by Canoe Circle Graphics
Editing by Karen Knox
Cover photo by Kristen Scott Photography
Bio headshot and family photo by © Scott Lawrence
Photo editing by Lee Smith

Printed in the U.S.A.

Dedication

I dedicate this book to three very special people who inspire me daily.

My two children, Noah and Ella. You are the reason this wellness journey began so many years ago and the reason I continue to work every single day to be a better version of myself. I thank you for enduring the persistent morning smoothies and endless green food that has filled your unique childhood.

Also, to my husband, Brian, who enthusiastically welcomes each new recipe test session, encourages every spontaneous whim, and is proudly my biggest fan. I could not possibly have done this without your daily support and unwavering faith.

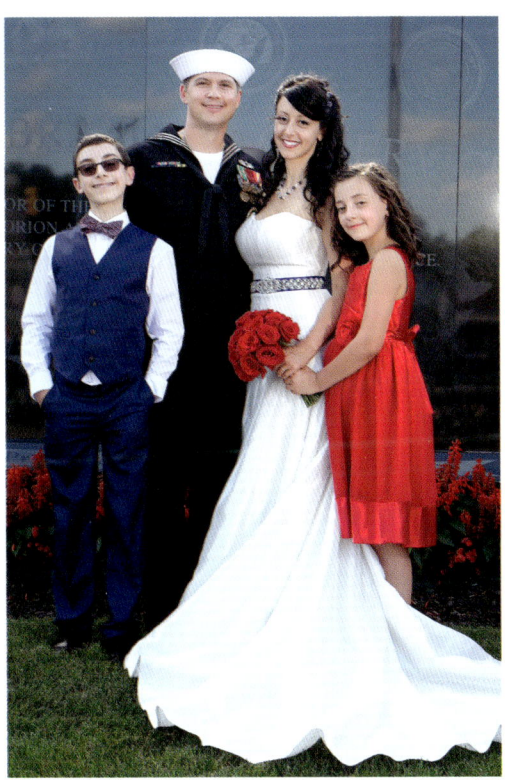

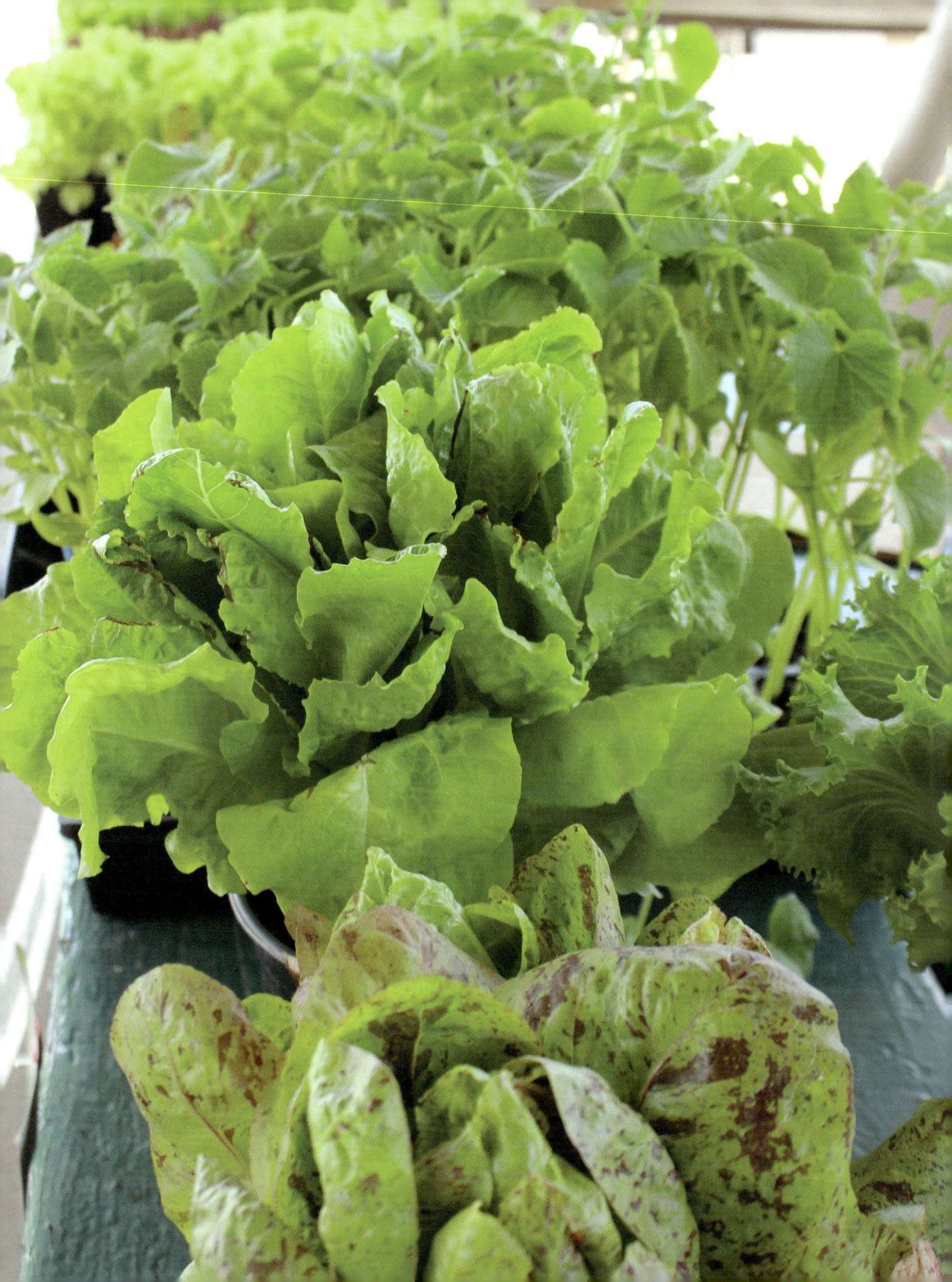

Table of Contents

As you make your way through this book, you may begin to notice that vegetables are often the star of the show. You will also find helpful tips along the way to ensure your journey is affordable, simple and of course—delicious! Here is your first tip: Do not throw away any veggie or fresh herb scraps. Check out the first recipe in the Supremely Dreamy Soups and Stews section and begin your broth collection with your very first recipe.

What is Holistic? 13

Recommended Supply List 17

Scrumptious Salads & Side Dishes 21

Supremely Dreamy Soups & Stews 43

Dee-Lish Dinners 65

Sensational Sauces & Spreads 87

Perfect Party Favorites 109

Satisfying Snacks & Sweets 131

About the Author 159

Acknowledgments 161

Additional Resources & Practitioners 163

Index By Ingredient 165

Index by Recipe Title 167

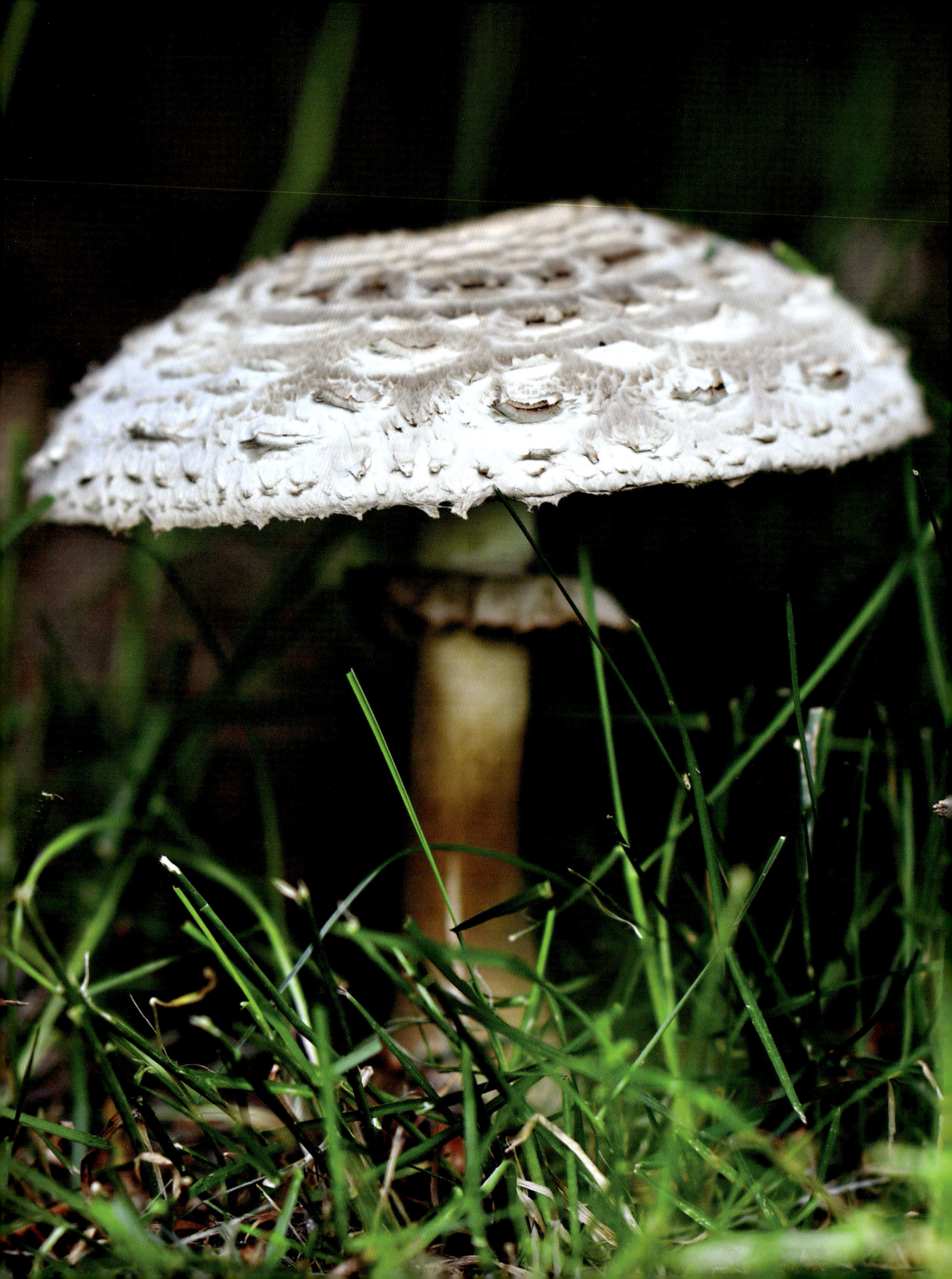

What is Holistic?

What is "holistic"? The term holistic comes from the word "whole" meaning—to be complete or in an unbroken, unaltered state. So much of today's world is a far cry from the original creation nature has supplied for us. Our bodies were designed to take in whole, natural food and clean, pure water. Since the standard American diet is made up of ingredients that no longer resemble these simple elements, disease and dysfunction have become the norm and food has become the enemy.

In my practice as a Nutritional Therapist, I repeatedly hear three reasons why folks are unable or unwilling to eat well:

- It's too expensive
- It's too difficult
- It doesn't taste good

In my efforts to debunk each of these, I began to host a series of cooking classes called Deliciously Holistic. At these classes, guests enjoy samples of three original recipes that are all affordable to shop for, simple to make, and taste incredible. Attendees were so inspired to get back into their kitchens and invest just a little time making real food again. I heard story after story about how their friends and family loved the dish, and how they couldn't wait until the next class. I had done it! I had inspired others to eat better for the benefit of their families and for themselves, and in turn, I was inspired to write this book.

Now it's your turn! But before you turn the oven on, let's take a moment to understand my philosophy and what type of food you can expect from this Deliciously Holistic home chef.

It's all about the love of real food. You will not find any corn starch or other processed ingredients in this book that look to cause harm in your body; only ingredients that began as food and still hold the same status by the time they reach your mouth are included. You also will not find any ingredients that are exceptionally expensive or impossible to find. Being well is not for the rich, it is for those who are mindful and willing to become a bit of a food snob like me. *(Like buying carrots with the tops still attached—snobby, I know).*

Each recipe is free from gluten, dairy, corn and refined sugars. If this was not simply a cook book I would expand on the reasons why those ingredients will never get near my fork. For more information on disease forming foods such as these, look to the resources page at the end of this book to find some of my favorite holistic-minded practitioners and medical professionals who all have written plenty for you to confidently learn from.

Lifelong wellness is never about counting the calories, the macros or any other scientific experiment—it is about being aware of the chemicals in your food and seeking out the most pure, unaltered form to fuel your body with. Choose organic whenever possible. When organic is not available, skip the packaged version of your produce and herbs and wash well with vinegar and water. Go for free-range,

Deliciously Holistic: Inspired Favorites

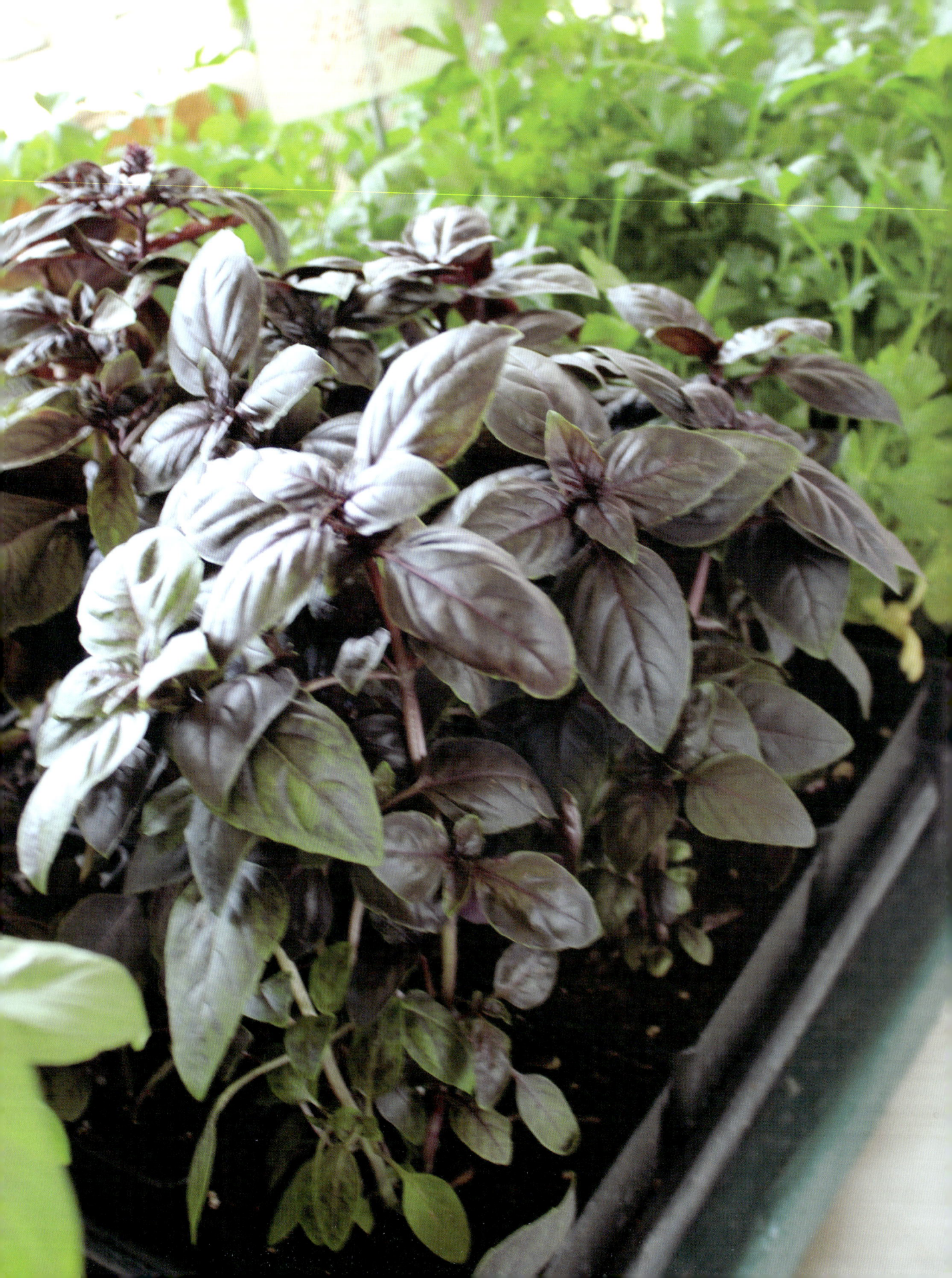

wild-caught and sustainably farmed labels wherever you can find them.

Every organ, tissue and cell are looking to be fed; fed with nutrients, sunlight, air and water. This must be why I am constantly seeking out any restaurant that offers outdoor dining, next to a body of water with the warm sun at my back. Not always the easiest task here in Michigan *(well the warm sun anyway)*, but an absolute perfect way to enjoy a meal and appreciate all that nature has to offer for my continued wellness.

Eat for color. Eat for variety. Eat from a reputable source, and eat food that still looks like food. Eat Well to Be Well, my friends.

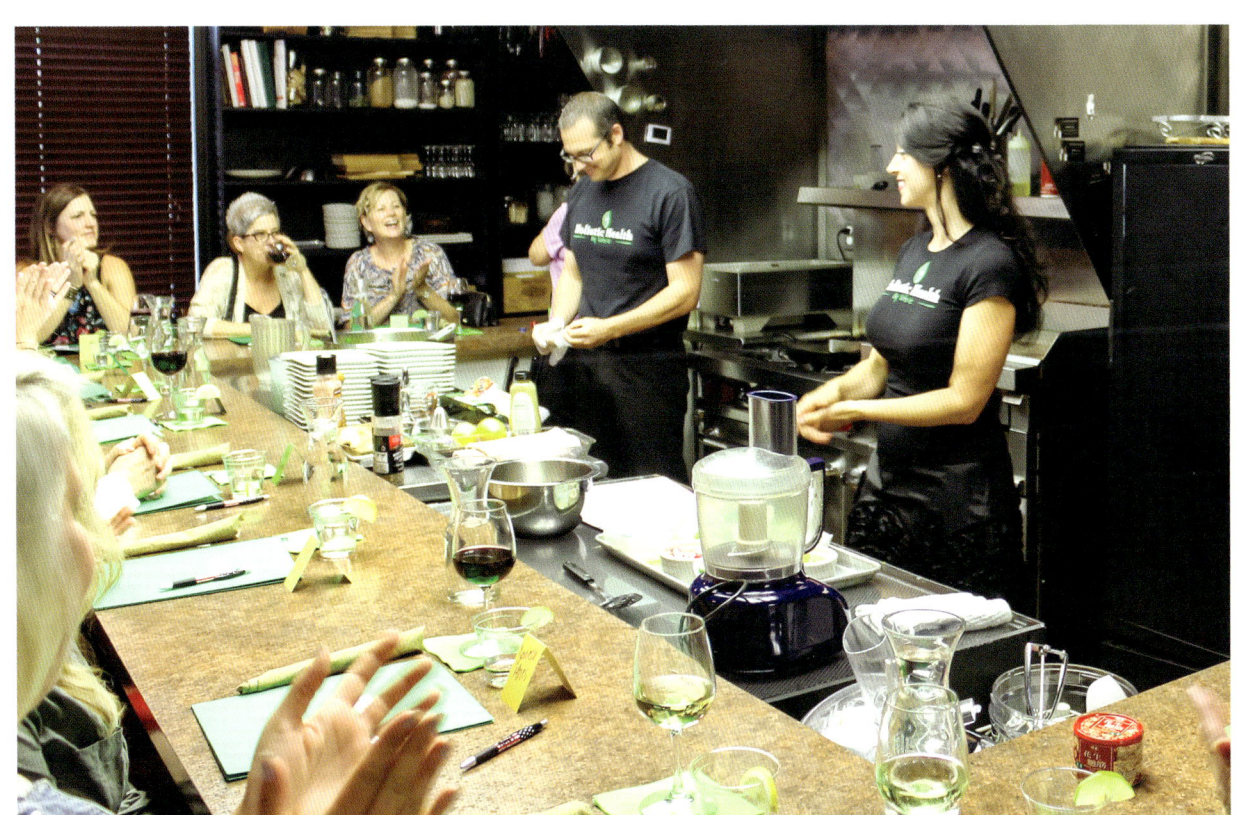

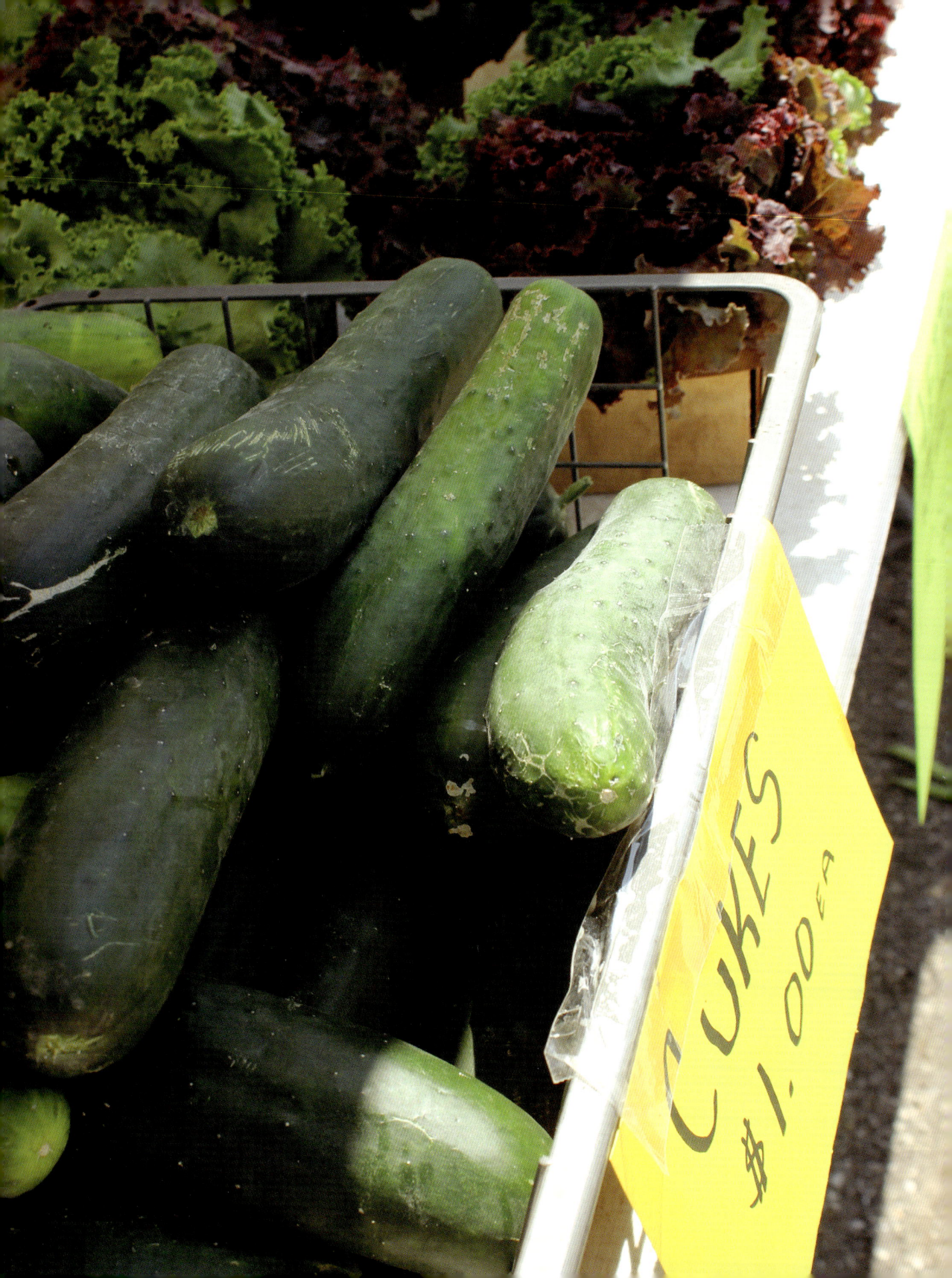

Recommended Supply List
FOR THE DELICIOUSLY HOLISTIC HOME CHEF

Nothing is more frustrating than getting half way through a recipe and realizing you do not have everything you need on hand to execute it as written. Although every recipe I create lends the opportunity to improvise, there are some common items you will never want to run out of. If you have never bought chia seed or coconut flour before, you may think it will be too expensive or tough to find. Fear not! The clean eating revolution is well underway and these items are now readily available almost everywhere. Even the large warehouse stores have jumped aboard the health trend train, so go ahead and buy the larger sized ingredient which brings down your cost per ounce. If you are often cooking for one, find a like-minded friend who is willing to split large packaged ingredients with you to keep your supply fresh.

- ☐ Nutritional yeast
- ☐ Liquid aminos or tamari (*gluten-free soy sauce*)
- ☐ Almond and coconut flour
- ☐ Array of fresh and dried herbs
- ☐ Array of tree nuts (*cashews, walnuts, pecans, almonds*)
- ☐ Pure maple syrup and raw honey (*the best stuff is at your local farmers market*)
- ☐ Himalayan sea salt

- ☐ Black pepper grinder (*fresh is always best!*)
- ☐ Cold-pressed avocado oil
- ☐ Raw, unrefined coconut oil
- ☐ Cold-pressed olive oil for cold and room temperature dishes only (*olive oil begins to lose its nutritional integrity when heated at high temperatures*)
- ☐ Unbleached parchment paper

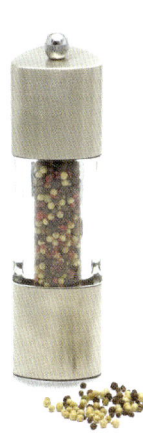

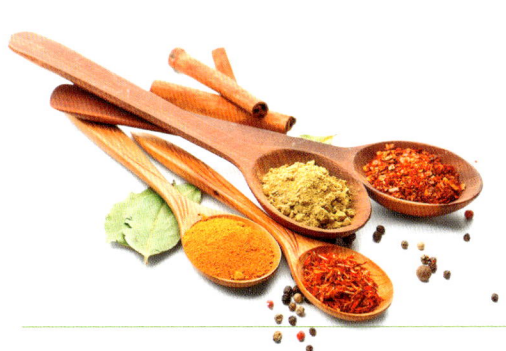

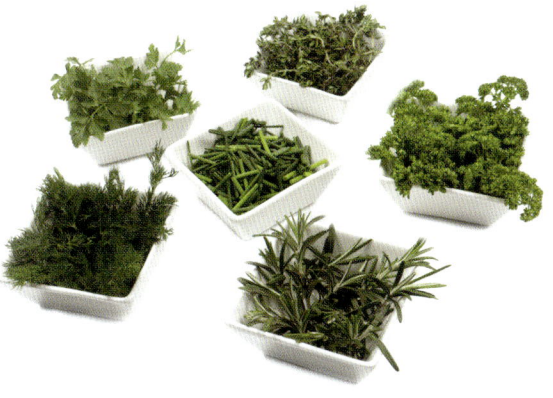

Deliciously Holistic: Inspired Favorites

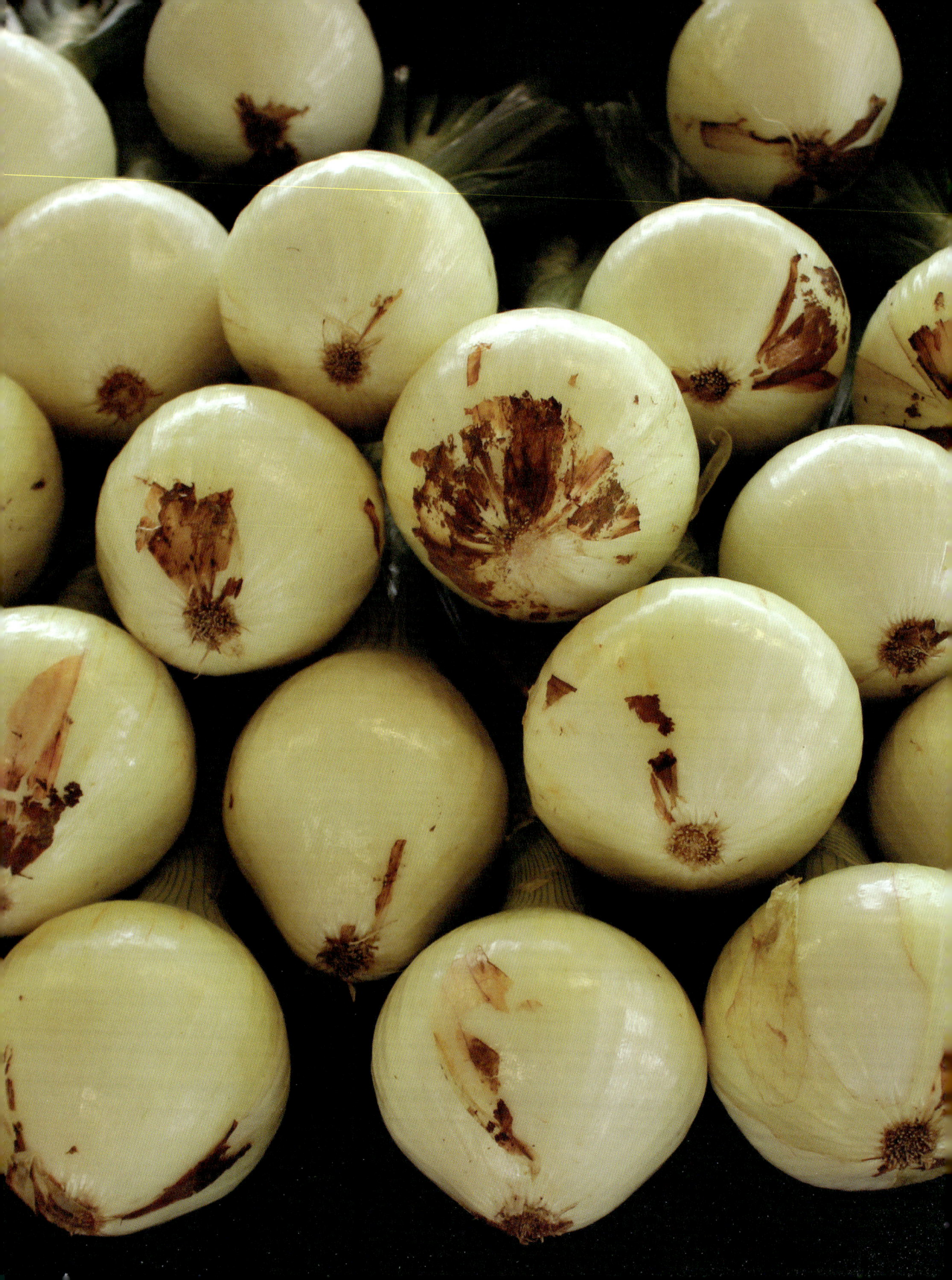

Recommended Supply List CONTINUED

FOR THE DELICIOUSLY HOLISTIC HOME CHEF

In addition, I recommend you obtain a few kitchen gadgets to make your culinary experience as effortless as possible. Remember, I promised your Deliciously Holistic experience would be simple, affordable and of course—delicious. The items below will help to keep me at my word.

- ☐ Cast iron pan(s) *(time to replace the Teflon please)*
- ☐ Glass or ceramic baking pans including a muffin tin
- ☐ Enamel-coated, cast-iron Dutch oven *(that's just a fancy name for a big ol' pot with a lid that can be used on the stove top or in the oven)*

- ☐ Array of wooden spoons *(ditch the plastic utensils)*
- ☐ Good quality chef's knife *(there's plenty of chopping in these recipes)*

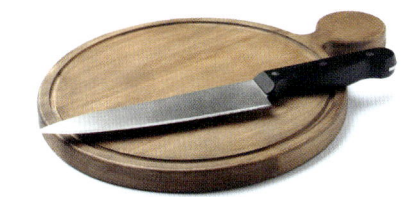

- ☐ Immersion blender
- ☐ Slow cooker
- ☐ Food processor
- ☐ Zester
- ☐ Kitchen blender

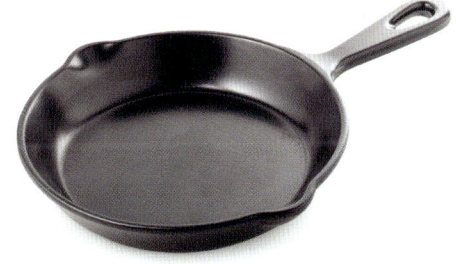

Deliciously Holistic: Inspired Favorites

Scrumptious Salads & Side Dishes

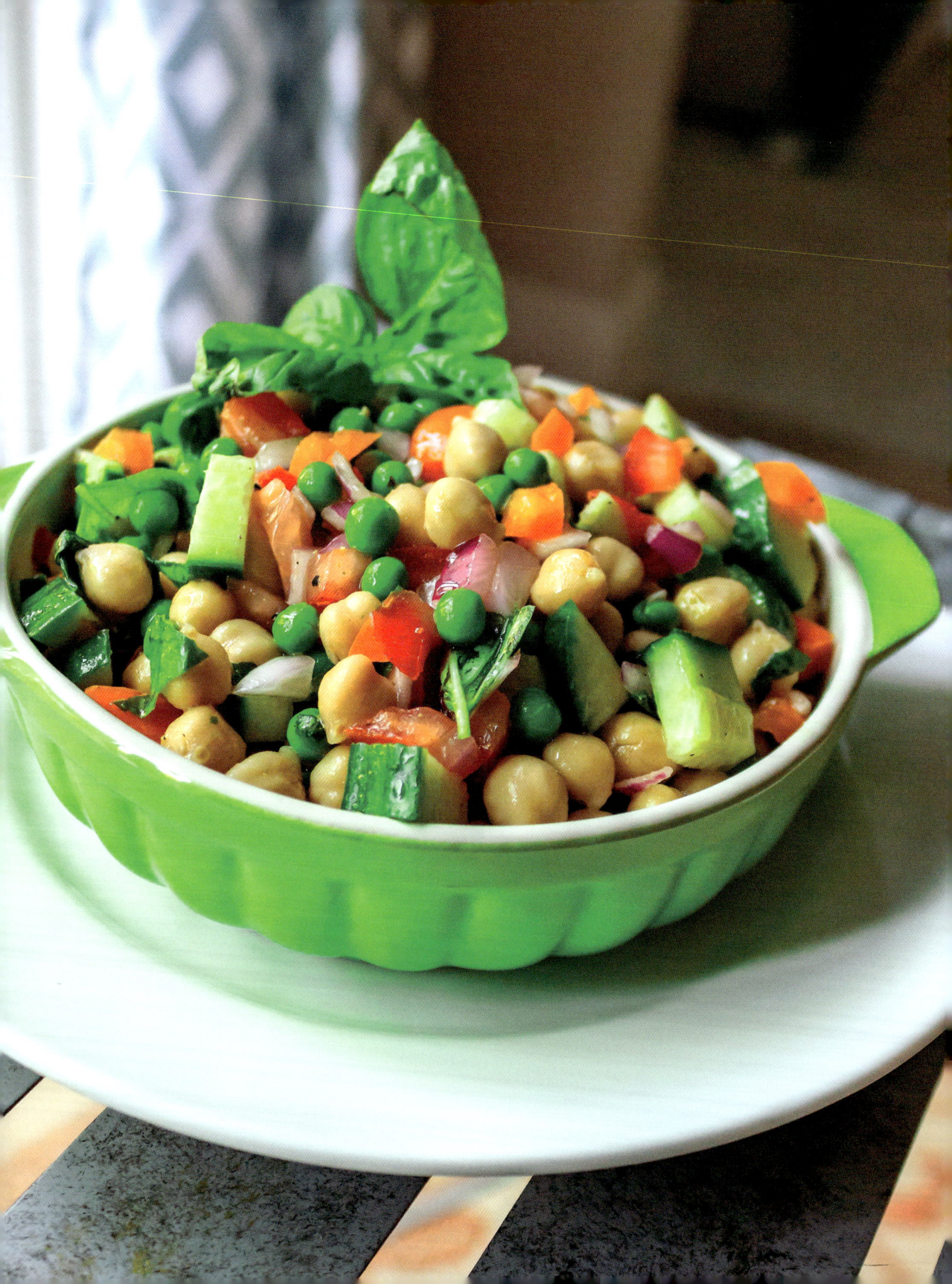

Pleasing Pea Salad

Not every salad needs to begin with lettuce. This recipe came out of a desire to create a summer side dish that could function as a salad, but would not look limp after a few hours of sitting in warm temperatures. It also features all of my favorite home garden veggies making it the most affordable dish of the season. Summers are meant for simple, fresh, and flavorful meals that take as little of your time away from the fun as possible.

1 *(15-ounce)* **can organic chickpeas, drained and rinsed**

1 cup green peas *(can be previously frozen)*

1 cup cucumber, diced

½ cup bell pepper, diced

½ cup red onion, diced

½ cup Roma tomatoes, diced and seeded

½ cup fresh basil, chopped

Juice from ½ lemon

1 tablespoon red wine vinegar

¼ cup olive oil

Sea salt and black pepper, to taste

Toss all ingredients together in a large bowl and serve with a smile to any crowd.

The flavor will get even better over time so if you are hoping for some leftovers, you may wish to make a double batch and scoop yourself a portion to hide in the back of the fridge.

Deliciously Holistic: Inspired Favorites

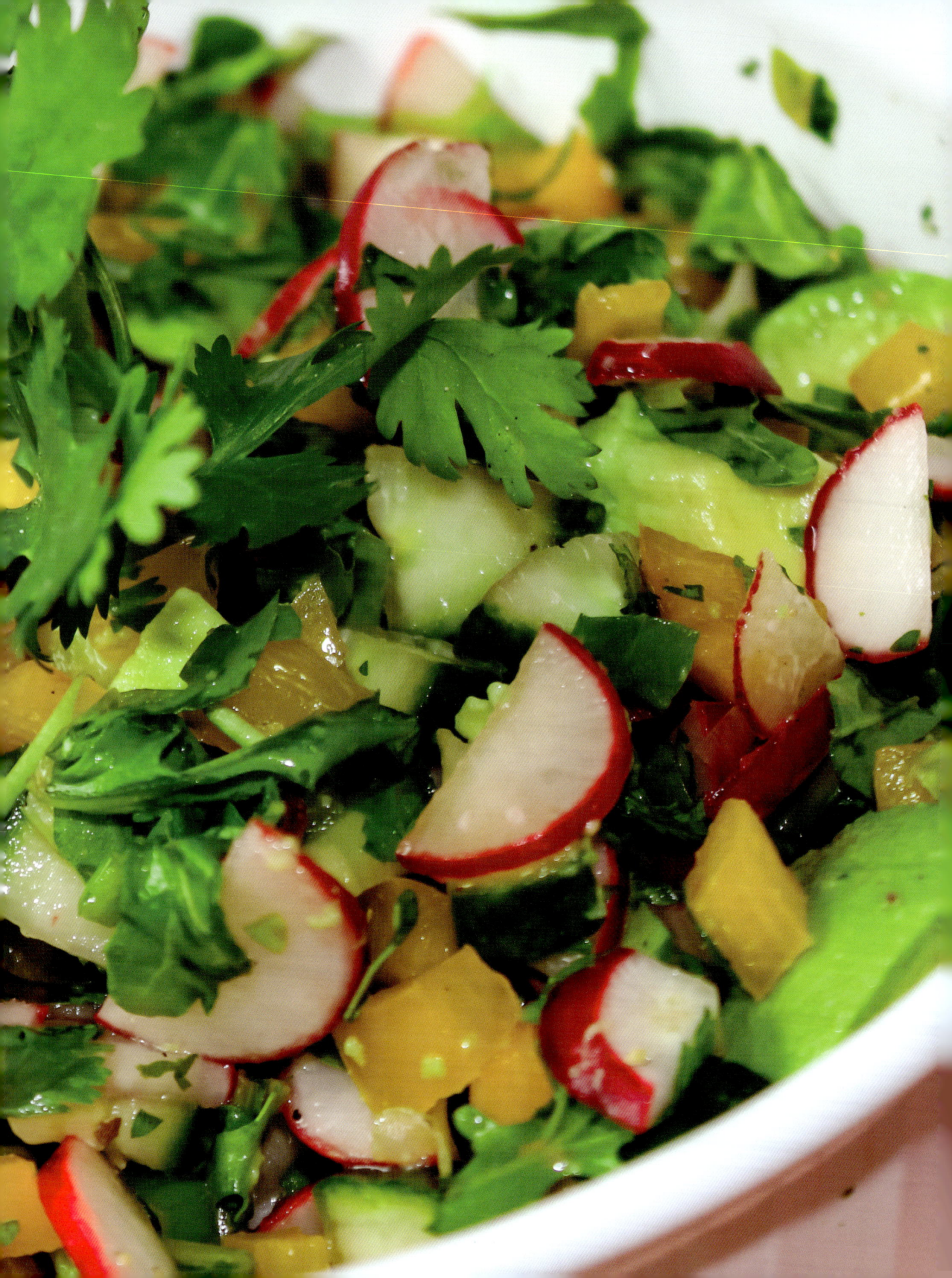

Cleansing Radish Ceviche

This recipe is bursting with cleansing nutrition because sometimes you just have to clean house! As a kid, I remember my dad would keep radishes in a bowl of water in the fridge and eat them whole as if he were eating candy. Now that I know how naturally detoxifying radishes are, I understand what a tremendous thing he was doing for his body. The great thing about the human body is that you don't necessarily need to be aware of how incredible a food is in order to reap the benefits. Your body knows exactly what to do with it; all you have to do is eat. Although my dad may not be excited about learning the science of nutrition, he is always excited about eating delicious food. Fortunately for him, his daughter cares about both.

10 radishes, thinly sliced

1 yellow bell pepper, petite diced

2 cups English (seedless) cucumber, petite diced

2 green onions, chopped

½ cup arugula, chopped

1 cup fresh cilantro, chopped

Juice from ½ lemon

Juice from 1 lime

1 avocado, diced

Sea salt and black pepper, to taste

Toss all ingredients in a large bowl except the avocado. Give the mixture a taste test and add more citrus juice or sea salt and black pepper if necessary. Gently fold in the avocado, keeping the pieces intact. You are not making guacamole and don't want to end up with mashed avocado.

For the best flavor, allow the ceviche to rest in the fridge for an hour before serving. Pairs perfectly with some Cajun spiced shrimp that has been seared on a hot grill. If the recipients are anything like my dad, feel free to skip the explanation of how beautifully detoxifying this dish is as they will be happily preoccupied with the party happening in their mouths.

Deliciously Holistic: Inspired Favorites

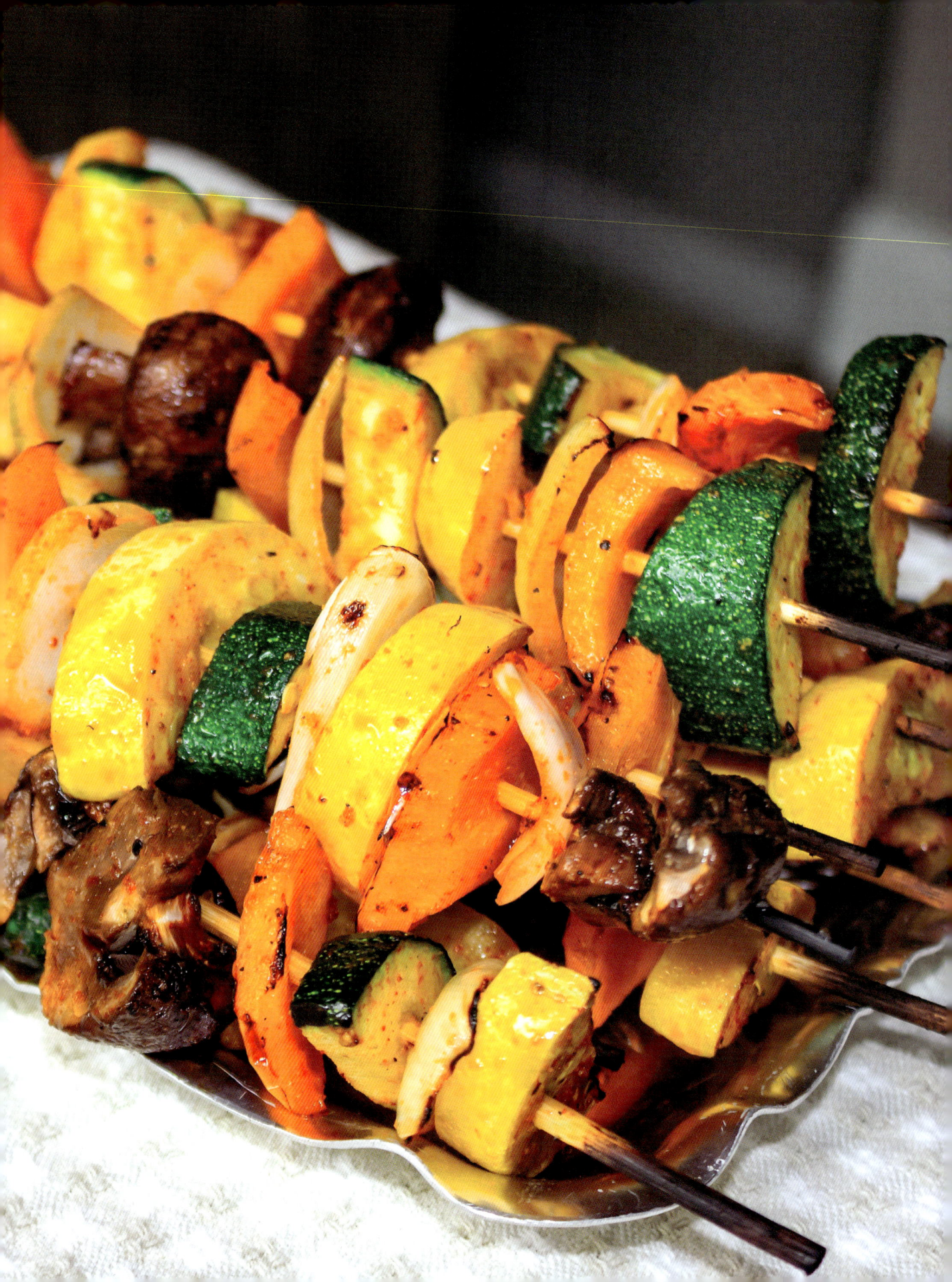

Veggie Skewers on the Barbie

You don't need to be an Aussie to enjoy throwing your meal "on the barbie" every now and then. As soon as the snow melts here in Michigan, I begin to crave the outdoors and seek every reason to soak up a little sun. Even vegetables seem to fit in with warm weather fun when they are stuck on a skewer and have a delightful barbeque flavor.

- **2 zucchini, cut into ½-inch slices**
- **2 yellow squash, cut into ½ inch slices**
- **1 large onion, chopped into bite-sized pieces**
- **1 bell pepper, chopped into bite-sized pieces**
- **8 ounces mushrooms, cut lengthwise in half**
- **2 tablespoons avocado oil**
- **1 teaspoon garlic powder**
- **1 teaspoon smoked paprika**
- **Sea salt and black pepper, to taste**

Preheat your grill to medium heat. Place all veggies in a large bowl and toss with the avocado oil, garlic powder, smoked paprika, sea salt and black pepper. Alternately thread all veggies onto wooden skewers. Cook for 3–4 minutes per side.

Pairs perfectly with chicken, steak, or seafood. If you are looking for a vegan meal, simply place your grilled veggies atop a pile of leafy greens and sprinkle with sliced almonds.

Tip: Although most grill masters would cringe to hear me say this, make sure to rotate your veggies and all grilled foods often; those traditionally sought-after grill marks are actually not good for your health and should be avoided.

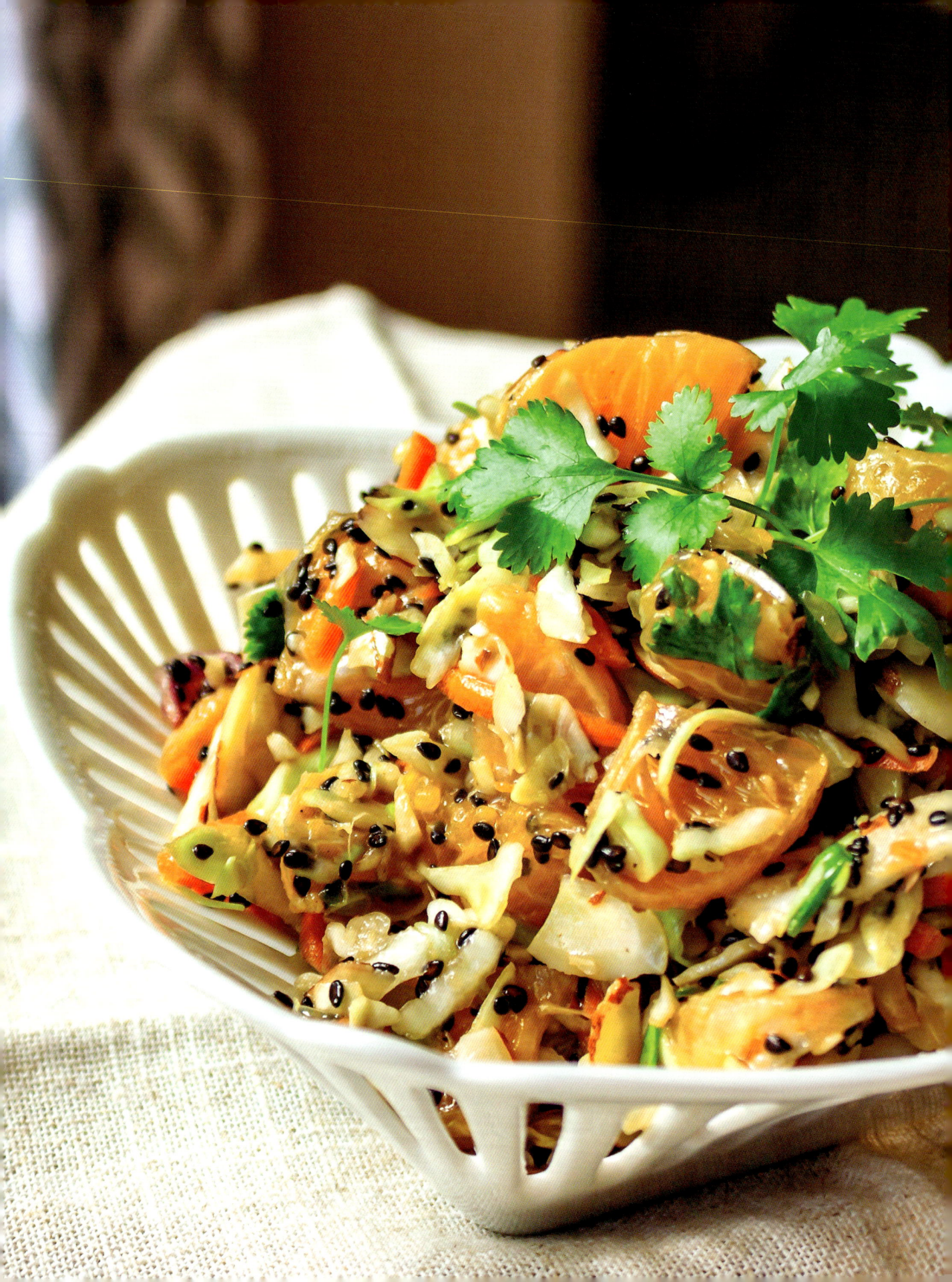

Vacation at Home Asian Slaw

I can never decide what I like best about this dish: the crunch, the colors, or the big, bright flavors. They are all equally satisfying. If you examine this recipe close enough, you will find it is essentially raw vegetables in a marinade. However, served alongside some grilled shrimp or scallops, you suddenly feel like you are on a vacation overseas. Quite honestly, if you were to travel outside of the great U. S. of A., more often than not you would find that international flavors are really about freshness and simplicity; the quality of the food speaks for itself. No preservatives or other unnecessary junk required (or requested for that matter). We can learn a lot from other cultures simply in the way they eat. Give this recipe a try and enjoy eating like you are on vacation without leaving the comfort of your own kitchen.

1 pound *(about 5 cups)* **rainbow slaw***

1 ½ cup sliced almonds

¼ cup sesame seeds

1 cup green onion, chopped

1 cup fresh cilantro leaves

4 mandarin oranges, peeled and broken into segments

*A rainbow slaw may include any of the following: red and green cabbage, carrot, broccoli and even cauliflower. Feel free to use any or all to create your favorite combination. You may buy pre-sliced or grab your favorite knife and slice everything yourself.

Dressing

¼ cup olive oil

2 tablespoons tamari or liquid aminos *(gluten-free soy sauce)*

2 tablespoons rice or white wine vinegar

1 tablespoon raw honey

1 tablespoon fresh ginger root, peeled and grated

Sea salt and black pepper, to taste

Combine all slaw ingredients in a large bowl and proceed to make the dressing.

Combine all dressing ingredients in a mason jar and shake well. Drizzle the dressing over the entire salad and toss until every bite is well coated.

Flavors will develop the longer you let it sit in the refrigerator; overnight is perfect, but certainly not required.

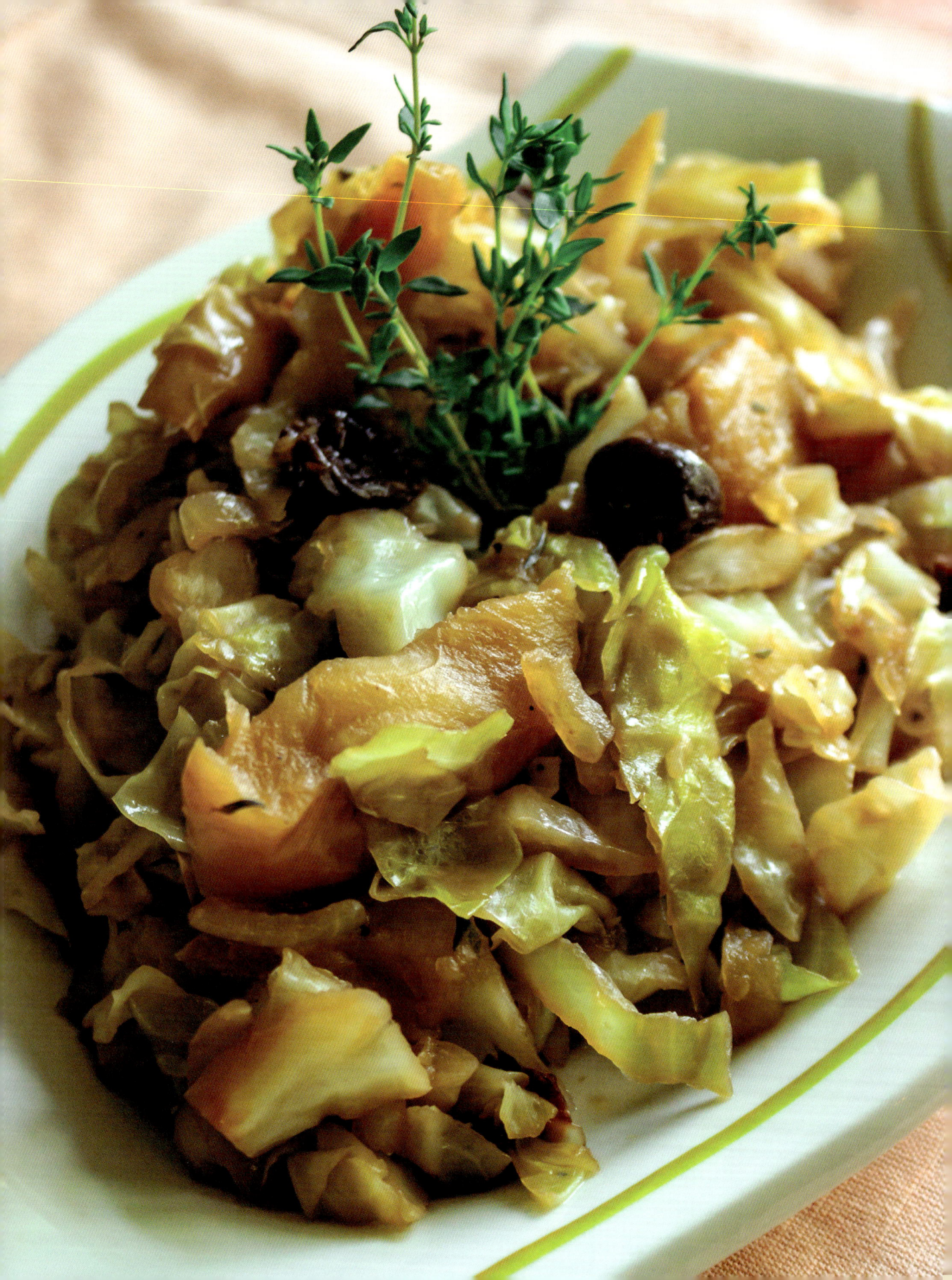

Savor your Sunday with Braised Cabbage and Apples

To me, Sundays are sacred. It is a day that should be devoted to resetting, rebalancing and relaxing from the week behind. Since part of what gives me joy is filling my kitchen with aromas that can only come from cooking real food, devoting part of the day to doing just that is exactly what I need to remember what is truly important. Savor your Sundays and allow this recipe to feed every bit of you that is in need of some love and attention.

1 teaspoon coconut oil

1 medium yellow onion, sliced

2 garlic cloves, chopped

1 tablespoon fresh thyme leaves

Sea salt and black pepper, to taste

3 apples, cored and cut into wedges

½ cup dried cherries *(look for the kind with no added sugar or simply organic fruit juice added)*

1 ½ cups vegetable broth

1 head green cabbage, thinly sliced or shredded

Heat coconut oil over medium heat in a large cast iron pot or Dutch oven. Add onion and sauté for 3–5 minutes until the onions start to look soft. Stir in the garlic, thyme, sea salt and black pepper and sauté for 1 minute.

Next add the apples, cherries and broth and stir to combine all ingredients. Finally, fold in the cabbage, cover the pot and place in the oven. Cook for 40 minutes until everything is soft and aromatic.

Serve alongside some pork chops for a hearty Sunday night dinner and forget all about the busy week ahead. Spend the evening connecting with your family or your very best friend and enjoy some genuinely good food that will feed your soul—and theirs.

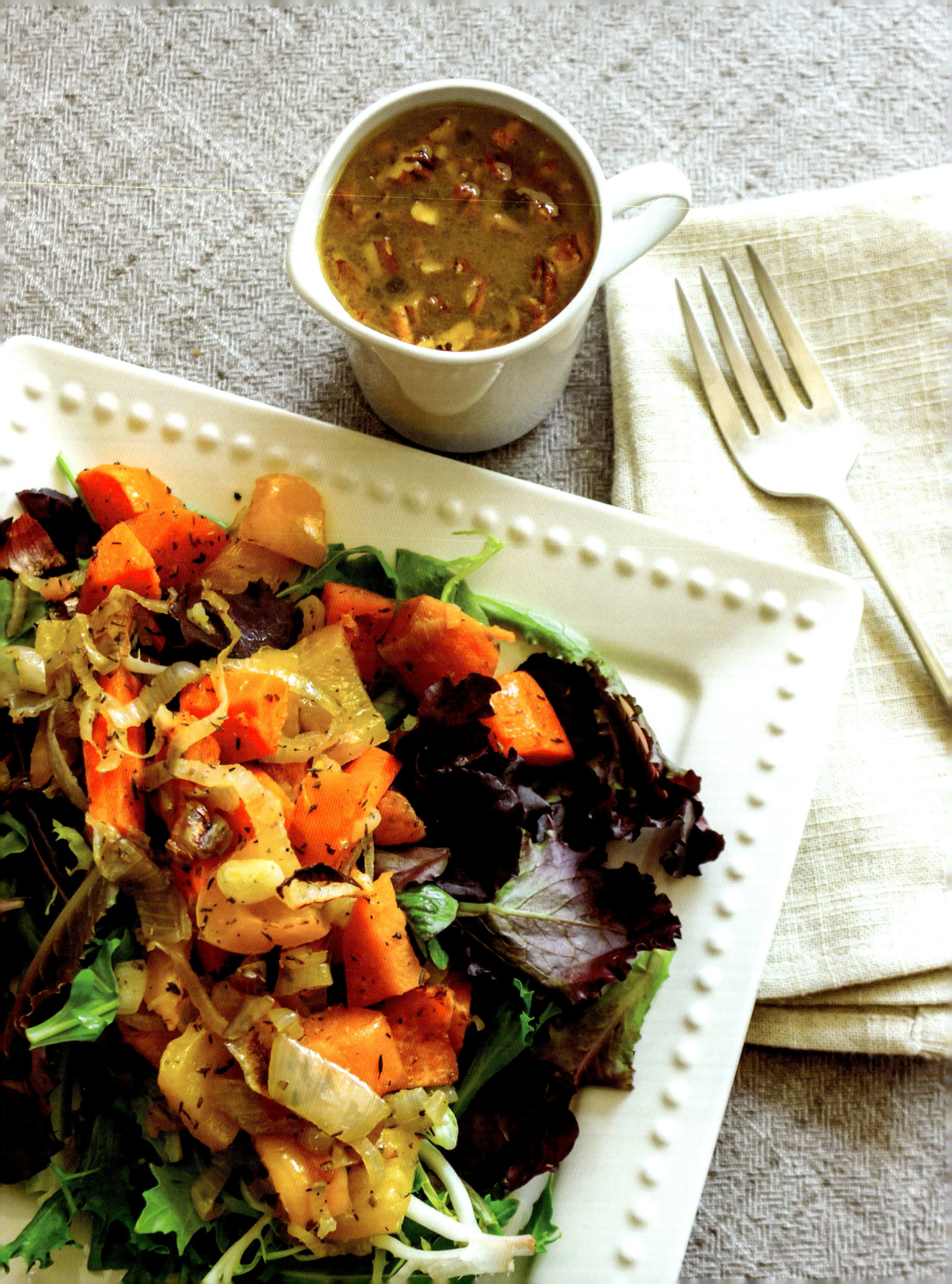

Roasted Veggie Salad with Warm Maple Pecan Vinaigrette

For many, a salad is what you eat before the real meal arrives. It might be what you opt for when you are watching your weight or trying to be polite on a date—"I'll just have a salad." This recipe proves that a salad can be so much more. It is every bit as satisfying as any restaurant quality entrée and is worthy of a spot on your dinner table.

1 medium sweet potato, peeled and cut into 1-inch chunks

1 large carrot, peeled and cut into 1-inch chunks

1 yellow bell pepper, cut into 1-inch pieces

2 shallots, sliced

Enough leafy greens to generously fill 2–4 dinner plates

1 tablespoon avocado oil

½ teaspoon dried thyme

½ teaspoon dried oregano

Sea salt and black pepper, to taste

Vinaigrette

½ cup avocado oil

¼ cup pure maple syrup

1 tablespoon apple cider vinegar

2 tablespoons Dijon mustard

½ cup pecans, finely chopped

Sea salt and black pepper, to taste

Preheat oven to 400 degrees. Place veggies in a glass baking dish and drizzle on the avocado oil, thyme, oregano, sea salt and black pepper. Be sure to use a big enough pan so that the veggies are not piled on top of each other. Toss well to coat. Place in the oven to roast for 30 minutes.

Add all vinaigrette ingredients to a small sauce pan and warm over low heat for 4–6 minutes. Stir occasionally.

Place a generous pile of mixed leafy greens onto your plate and top with roasted veggies. Finish with a generous drizzle of your warm maple pecan vinaigrette.

Did you ever think a salad could be so decadent? Welcome to the delicious world of eating well!

Deliciously Holistic: Inspired Favorites

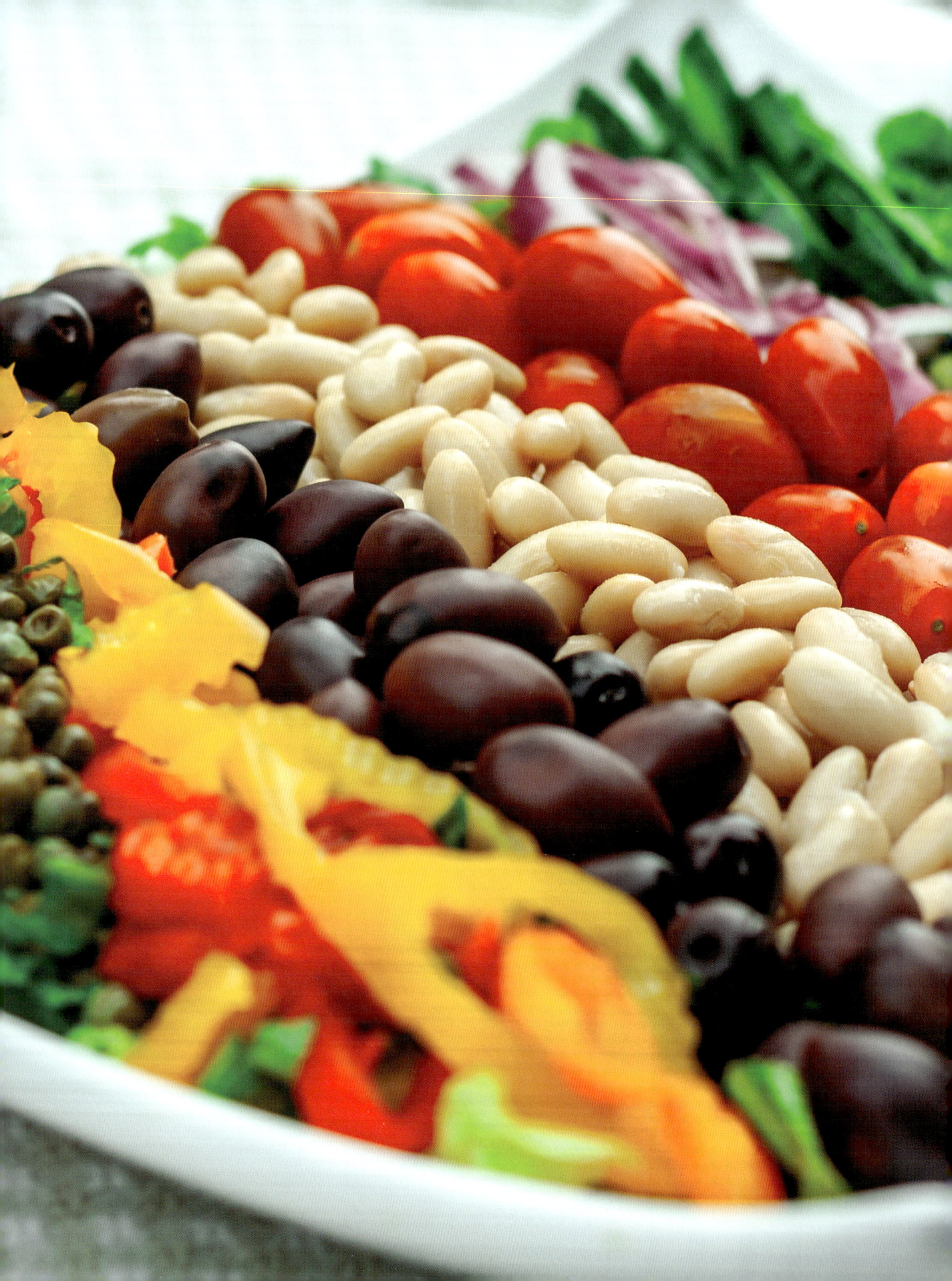

"I'll Bring the Salad" Salad

We tend to enjoy food with our eyes long before it greets our stomachs. Even something as simple as a dinner salad can be made to visually entice our taste buds. I was recently asked to "just bring the salad" to a large event and was surprised that the hostess did not take the opportunity to ask for something that required a little more effort. Certainly, she knows I teach cooking classes, right? After the event, she admitted to being afraid I would show up with some crazy vegan blob of healthy goo that no one would touch. When I arrived with this display of beautiful food it instantly became a conversation piece. Now, I always offer to bring the salad whenever anyone is having a potluck-style gathering; it requires very little effort, is exceptionally affordable to put together, and is very well received by all. Always offer to bring the salad, and enjoy being the hit of the party.

4–6 cups romaine lettuce, finely chopped

1 *(15-ounce)* can organic cannellini beans, drained and rinsed

1 small red onion, thinly sliced

1 orange or yellow bell pepper, thinly sliced

1 *(4-ounce)* jar capers, drained

1 cucumber, sliced on an angle

6 ounces Greek olives, pitted

8 ounces cherry or grape tomatoes

1 *(12-ounce)* jar pepperoncini

Balsamic or raspberry vinaigrette (with no added sugars)

Using a large platter, spread the romaine along the bottom. Next, create rows on an angle with each ingredient lined up to the next.

Place a bowl full of dressing on the side with a spoon and be sure to supply tongs for easy serving among guests.

Tip: You can easily swap out your toppings to design a unique salad every time. Try thinly sliced white button mushrooms, sun-dried tomatoes, pumpkin or sunflower seeds, dried cherries, pomegranate seeds, and thinly sliced pear. There's no limit to the flavor combinations you can create so have fun with it!

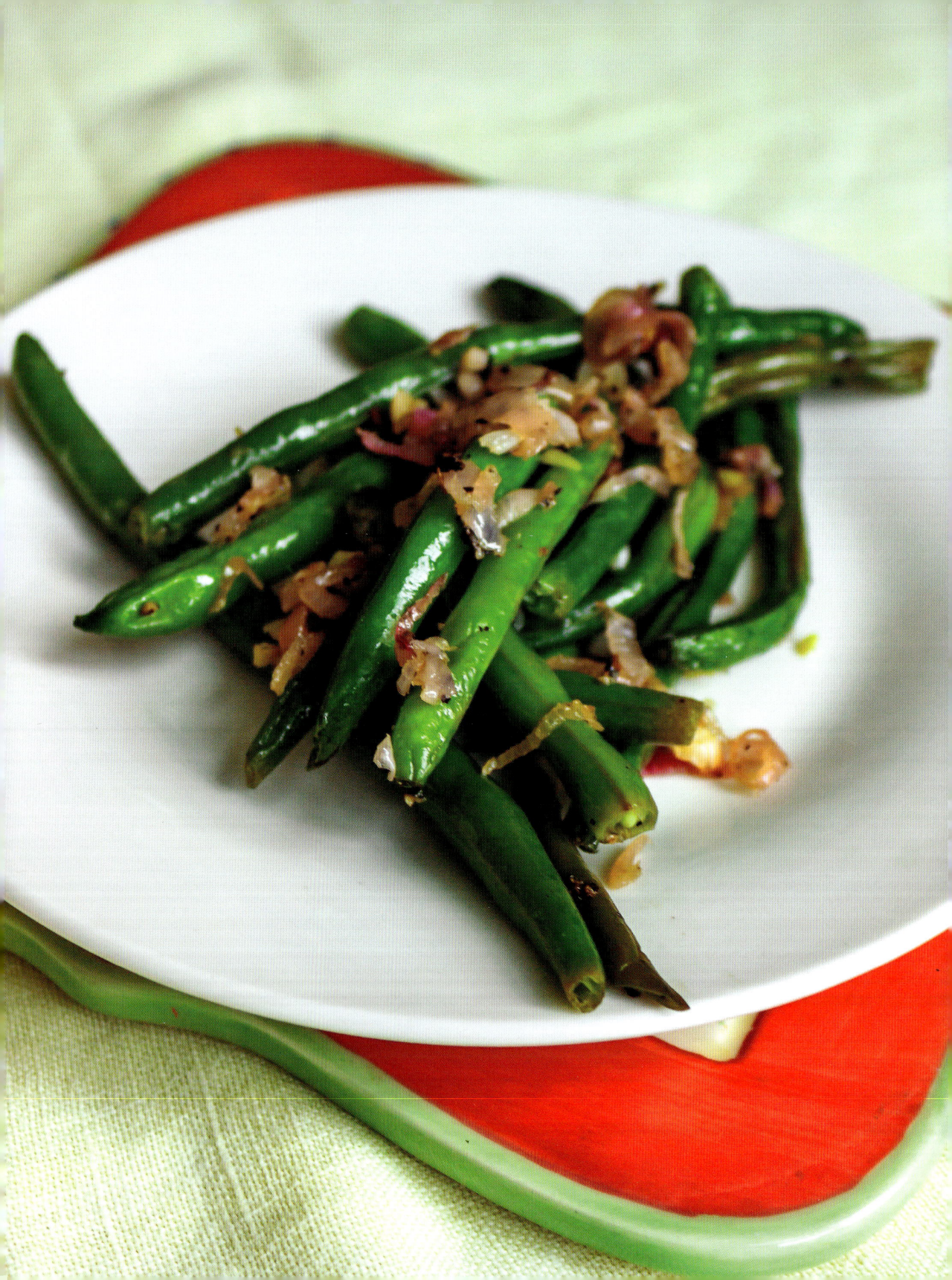

Grateful for Green Beans

Affordable, easy to find, and loved by all. Green beans are perhaps the most well-received green vegetable (yes broccoli, I am sure you are a close second) that could ever land on your dinner table. Whether you are serving these alongside a fancy filet mignon or a simple turkey wrap, they make for the perfect accompaniment. If you have previously been accustomed to using frozen or canned beans, please oh please try this recipe with fresh green beans. Your taste buds will certainly be grateful.

1 pound fresh green beans, trimmed

1 shallot, very thinly sliced

2 garlic cloves, very thinly sliced

1 tablespoon avocado oil

Juice from ½ lemon

Sea salt and black pepper, to taste

Preheat oven to 375 degrees. Add all ingredients to a glass or ceramic baking dish and toss well.

Place in the oven and cook for 8–10 minutes. Remove from the oven and give everything a good toss, then place back into the oven to cook for another 6–8 minutes.

Tip: As soon as you bring your beans home from the store, give them a rinse and a trim and store them in a bowl lined with paper towel until you are ready to use them. Having the prep work completed in advance makes putting dinner together exceptionally simple.

Deliciously Holistic: Inspired Favorites

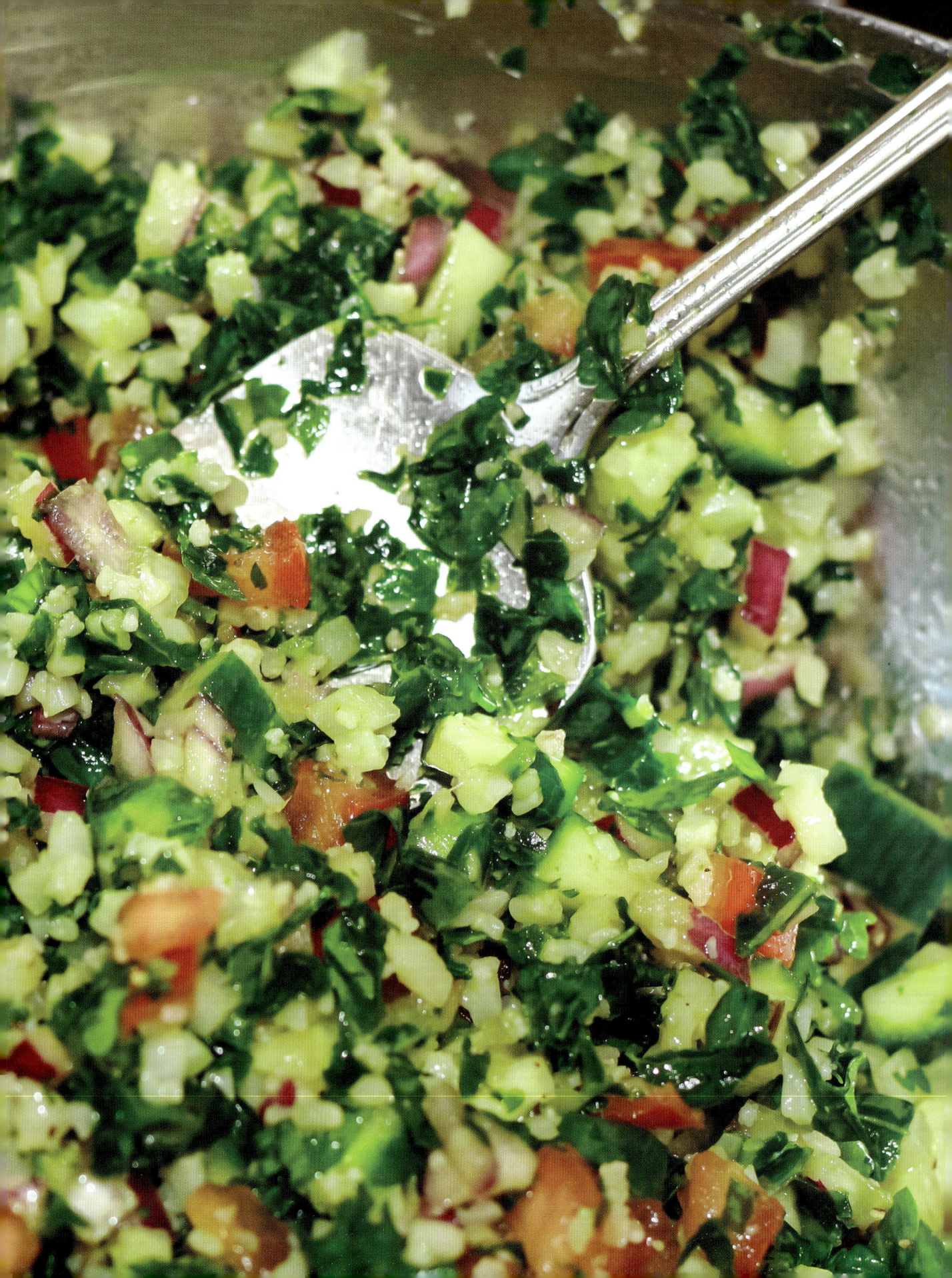

Traditional Tabbouleh with a Twist

One of the fondest memories from my childhood is when my grandmother would send me into her backyard to pick the fresh parsley that would be turned into tabbouleh for that evening's family dinner. If I were really lucky, she would allow me to pick the leaves from the stems and add them to the bowl. Her tabbouleh included bulgur wheat which I have replaced with riced cauliflower in order to keep it gluten-free. I have also added kale to make this exceptionally nutritious dish even more powerful. If she were still with us, I'm hopeful she would overlook my substitutions and acknowledge my efforts to honor her and our family traditions.

2 cups riced cauliflower *(I buy it frozen and thaw it overnight in the fridge)*

1 ½ cups seedless cucumber, petite diced

1 ½ cups flat Italian parsley, chopped

1 ½ cups kale leaves *(ribs removed)*, **finely chopped**

1 ½ cups tomato, seeds removed and diced

1 ½ cups red onion, petite diced

Juice from 1 lemon

¼ cup of olive oil

Sea salt and black pepper, to taste

Combine all ingredients in a large bowl and toss to combine. Flavors will develop over time but you can adjust the seasoning and amount of lemon juice according to taste.

Traditionally this dish should have a strong lemon flavor. It can be served at room temperature or chilled and makes a great side dish for any outdoor party.

If you really want to experience this dish the way I did as a kid, enjoy it with plenty of hummus and kibbee nayee. I'll save you the suspense and Google search—it's a traditional Lebanese dish made of raw lamb, and I still eat a ton of it!

Deliciously Holistic: Inspired Favorites

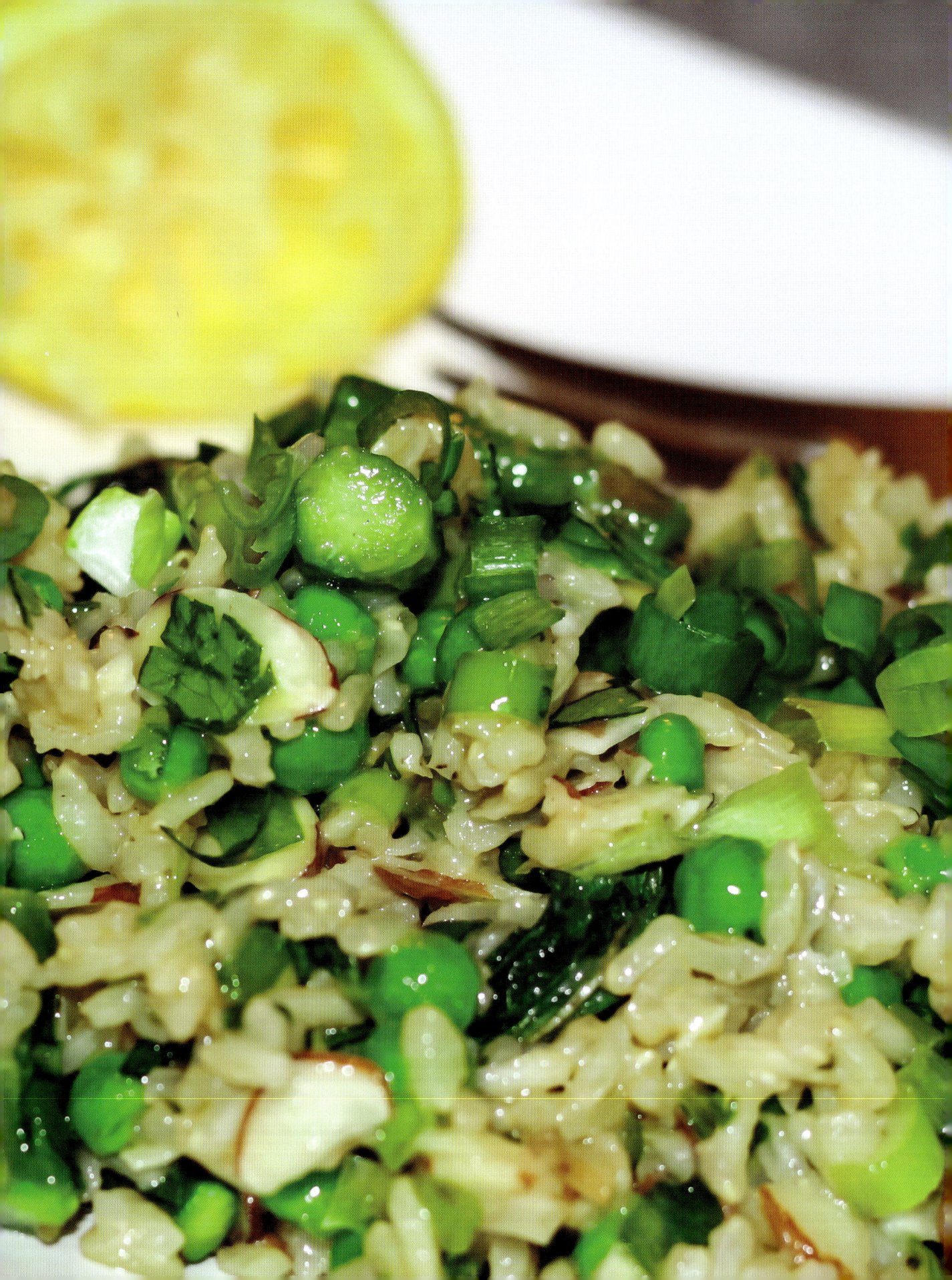

Herb Spring Salad with Jasmine Rice

When warm temperatures and longer days return with the coming of spring, all I want to do is get into my kitchen with fresh green ingredients to celebrate. This recipe is a wonderful reason to gather with friends and rejoice in all things new.

1 cup uncooked brown jasmine rice *(this will yield about 2 ½ cups of cooked rice)*

14–16 asparagus spears

½ tablespoon coconut oil

Sea salt and black pepper, to taste

¼ cup olive oil

1 cup green peas *(can be fresh out of the pod or previously frozen)*

½ cup sliced almonds

½ cup chopped green onion

⅓ cup fresh chopped cilantro

⅛ cup fresh chopped mint

Juice from ½ lemon

Make brown jasmine rice according to the instructions on the package. While the rice cooks, wash the asparagus and trim the ends. Dry with a paper towel and add the asparagus to a glass or ceramic baking dish. Lightly coat the asparagus with coconut oil and season with sea salt and black pepper. Place in a 400-degree oven to roast for 12–14 minutes until the asparagus is cooked but not mushy. Remove from the oven and allow to cool. Chop into bite sized pieces.

Once the rice is fully cooked, fluff with a fork and add it to a large bowl, allowing it to cool as well.

Next, add the asparagus, green peas, sliced almonds, green onion, cilantro, mint and lemon juice to the bowl. Toss with olive oil and more sea salt and black pepper until all ingredients are mixed well.

Serve at room temperature or chilled out of the refrigerator. Flavors will develop the longer they have to sit in the fridge so leftovers may be better than the original. Pairs nicely with some grilled shrimp or ahi tuna.

Tip: Instead of using water when making your rice, substitute a bone broth or vegetable stock to add flavor and nutrients. When buying store bought broth always ensure sugar is not listed as an ingredient. Even in the organic broths, sometimes they can sneak that ingredient by you.

Supremely Dreamy Soups & Stews

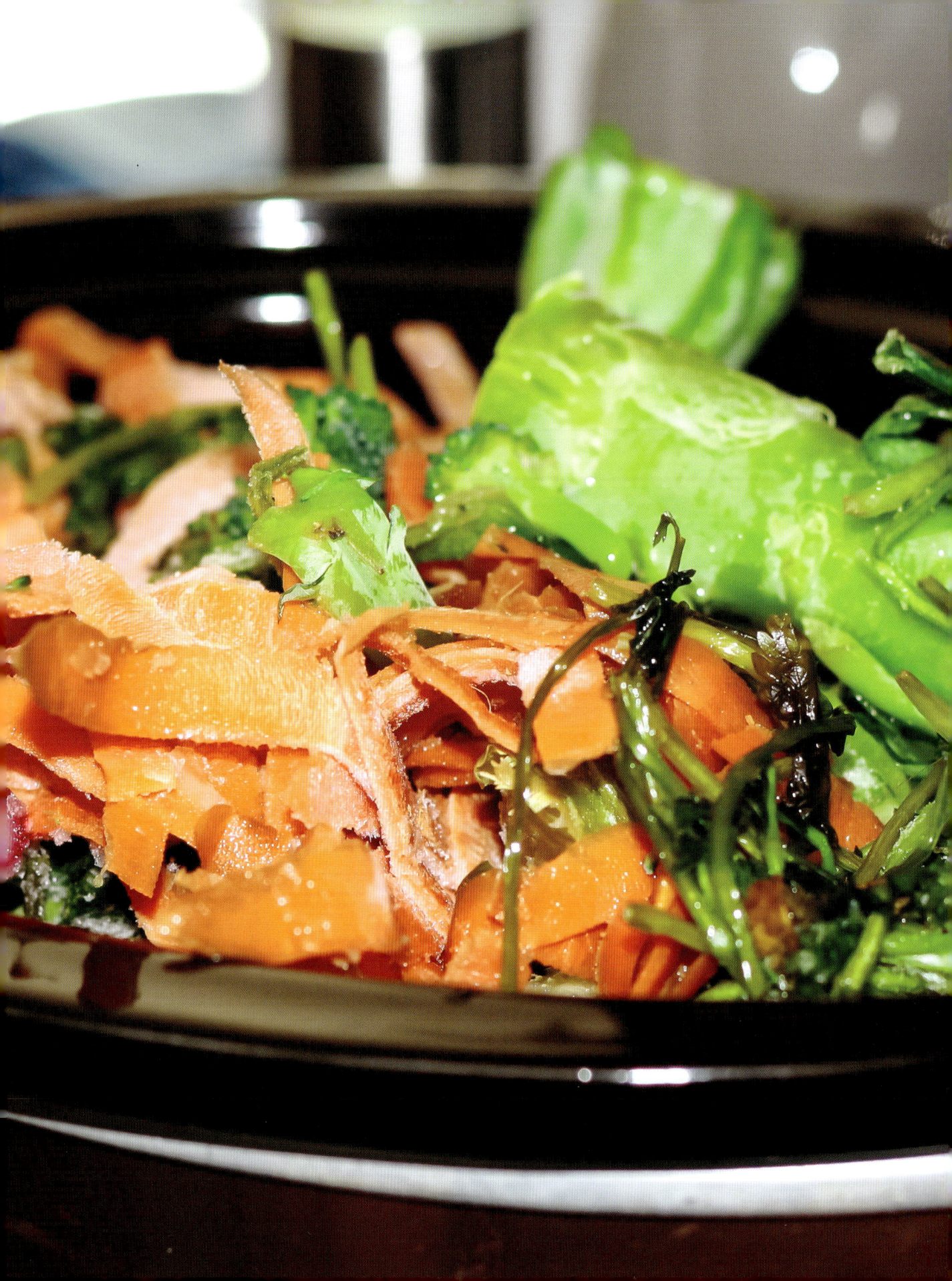

Waste not, Want not Vegetable Broth

Years ago, I worked in a little French styled bistro named Victoria's in Oxford, Michigan. The owner, Victoria Connolly is a big believer of making use of every single bit of food that enters her restaurant. I learned very quickly to never throw away the tops of a strawberry as she would be using them to make a flavored simple-syrup for a hand-crafted cocktail. Once I began to advise others on how to prepare mindful meals, I needed to make sure their shopping (and spending) efforts never went to waste. Making your own vegetable broth is simple and smart. Why throw away any bit of those organic veggies and fresh herbs when they could be the base of a delicious soup? This recipe is included in this book not only to save you some cash, but also to pay tribute to a lovely woman who taught me the art of "waste not, want not."

Keep all leftover veggies and fresh herbs that you would normally discard such as onion skin, pepper and carrot tops, celery and radish ends, parsley stems, broccoli stalks, etc. Anything that has color contains precious nutrients that you want to make use of in the form of a vegetable broth.

Ensure the leftovers are washed and place them in the freezer in a glass or ceramic container. Once you have enough to fill a slow cooker, place the frozen veggies/herbs in your pot and fill with enough water to cover the veggies. Put the lid on and set the temperature on low. Cook for a minimum of 6 hours or up to 12.

Allow to cool slightly and drain the liquid into glass jars. Store the broth in the fridge or freezer until you are ready to use. At this point the veggies should have lost all of their vibrant color and are now ready to be thrown away.

Broth that is stored in the refrigerator will remain fresh for 5-7 days and can be used in any recipe that calls for chicken, beef or vegetable broth. You can also use the broth instead of water when making rice or quinoa.

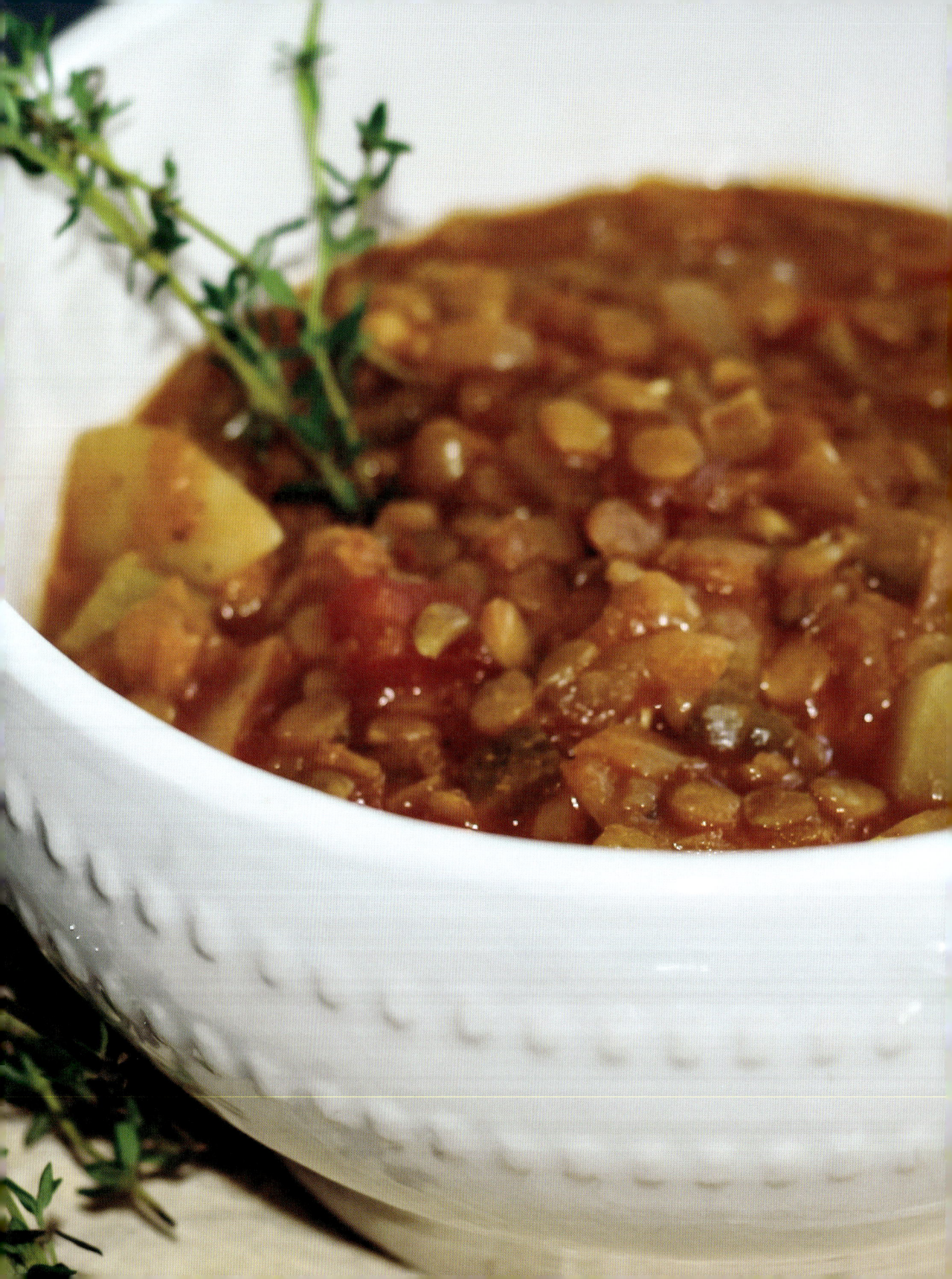

Hearty Lentil Stew

Depending on where you live, the winter can be a long and brutal season. However, these conditions regularly inspire me to create dishes that are warm and comforting. Since winter is the season for rest, feel free to double or triple this recipe so that you can easily freeze the leftovers and pull it out on those days that you are truly in need of some rest or recovery.

1 tablespoon coconut or avocado oil

1 yellow onion, chopped

1 large carrot, peeled and chopped

2 celery stalks, chopped

2 cloves garlic, minced

1 (15-ounce) can diced organic tomatoes

2 cups dried green or brown lentils

1 teaspoon sweet or smoked paprika *(depending on your preferred flavor)*

1 teaspoon ground cumin

1 tablespoon fresh thyme leaves OR ½ tablespoon dried thyme leaves

Sea salt and black pepper, to taste

4 cups vegetable stock or bone broth

2 medium-sized potatoes, diced *(Yukon gold or sweet potatoes)*

Heat the oil in a soup pot over medium heat. Add the onion, carrot and celery and cook until the vegetables are soft and tender, 6 to 8 minutes. Stir in the garlic and cook for 1 minute more.

Add the tomatoes, lentils, paprika, cumin, thyme and salt and pepper; stir well to incorporate all ingredients. Add the stock and potatoes and bring to a boil. Reduce the heat to maintain a simmer, cover the pot and continue cooking until the potatoes are tender.

Tip: *If you want an easy way to add some additional flavor to this soup, simply swap out 15 ounces of your favorite chunky salsa instead of using canned tomatoes.*

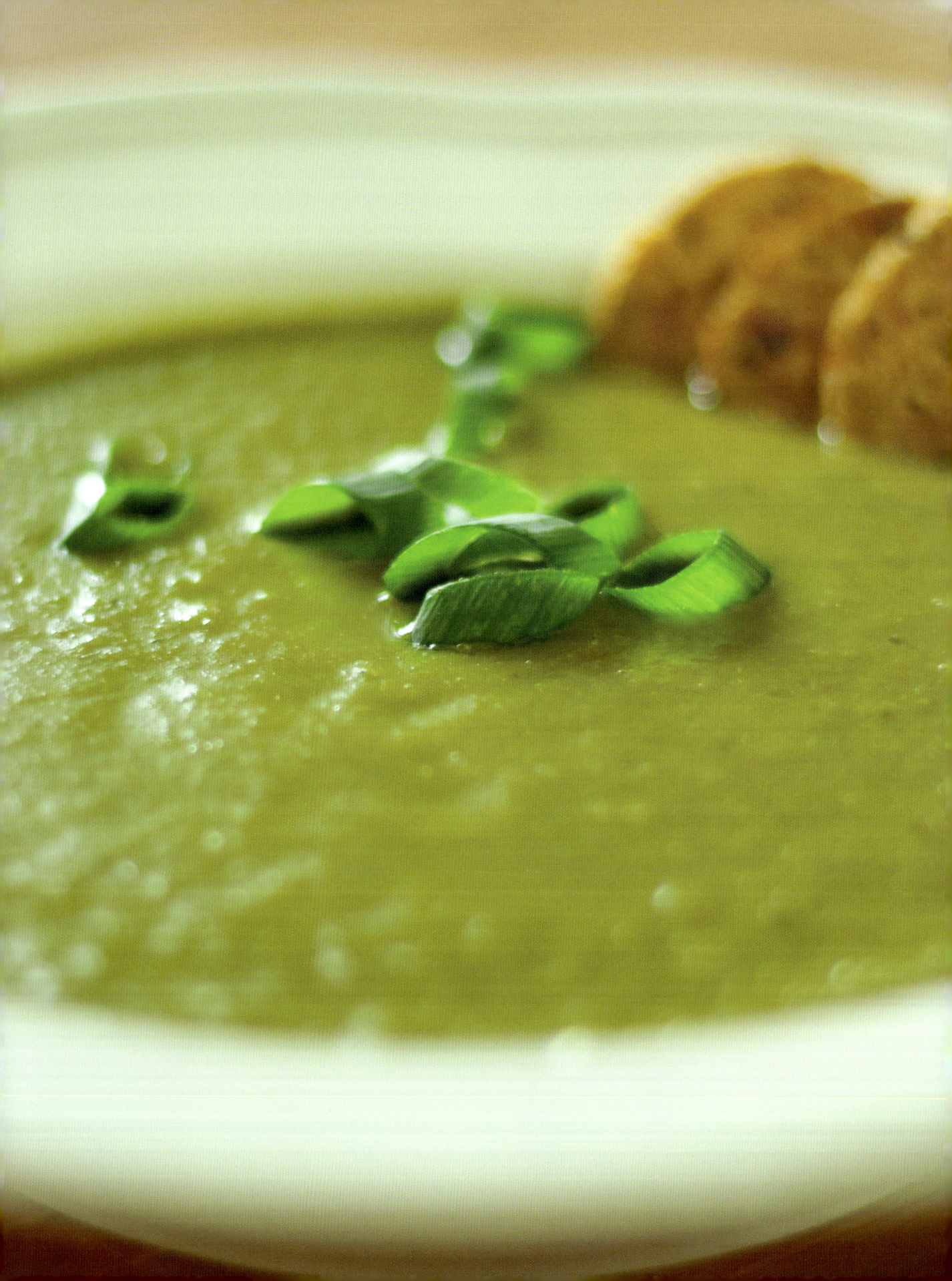

Creamy Asparagus Bisque FOR ANTI-ASPARAGUS FOODIES

My son is certainly a major foodie like his mom. Although we share a love of real food, there is one vegetable he always scowls at: asparagus. In my many attempts to showcase this statuesque green veggie in a palatable way, none had proved successful until this soup was placed before him. The secret to my success may be the flavor profile, the creamy consistency, or simply the means to eat his favorite crackers. But whatever the reason, I now confidently serve him asparagus and receive a "Thanks for dinner, Mom" in return.

- **1 tablespoon coconut oil**
- **1 medium yellow onion, chopped**
- **1 yellow bell pepper, chopped**
- **2–3 celery stalks, chopped**
- **1 garlic clove, chopped**
- **1 pound asparagus, trimmed and chopped into bite-sized pieces**
- **1 cup green peas** (*I advise against using canned; fresh or previously frozen is best*)
- **1 teaspoon dried or 1 tablespoon fresh thyme**
- **1 teaspoon dried or 1 tablespoon fresh oregano**
- **Sea salt and black pepper, to taste**
- **4 cups vegetable or chicken broth**
- **Hot sauce** (*optional*)
- **Gluten-free crackers** (*optional*)

In a large soup pot, melt coconut oil over medium heat. Add onion, bell pepper and celery and sauté until soft about 6–8 minutes. Stir in the garlic and cook for one minute more. Next add asparagus, peas, thyme, oregano, sea salt and black pepper and give another good stir to incorporate all ingredients. Add the broth and raise the heat to bring to a boil.

Once the soup is boiling, lower the heat to a simmer, cover with the lid and cook until the asparagus is soft, about 10–12 minutes.

Using an immersion blender, blend the soup until you achieve a creamy consistency. You can also blend the soup in batches in a blender to accomplish this if you do not have an immersion blender. Serve with gluten-free crackers for some added crunch and a few dashes of hot sauce.

Once you have fully embraced your new love for asparagus, get creative in the kitchen with your next under-admired vegetable.

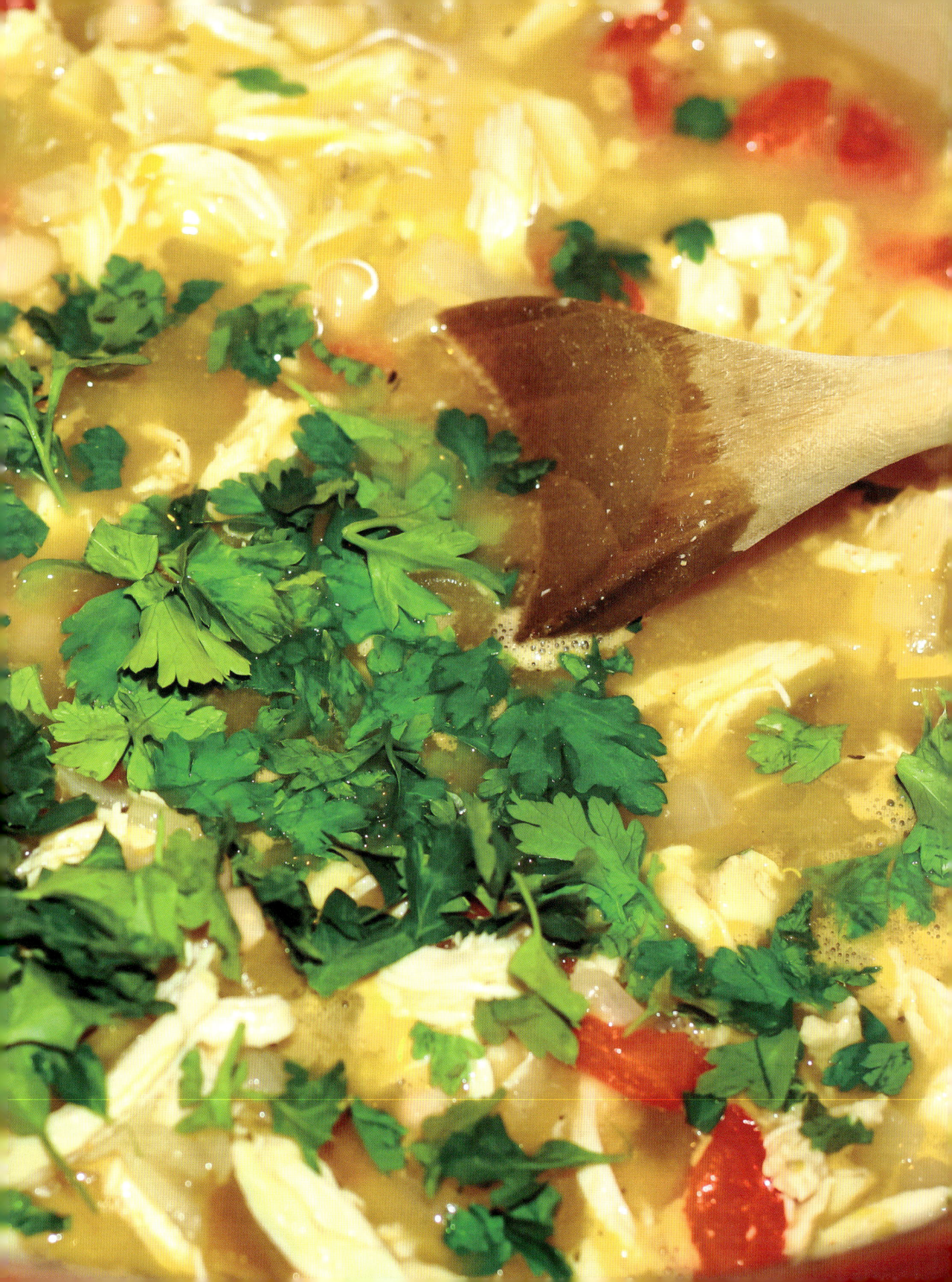

For the Love of Cumin Chicken Chili

Growing up, my Aunt Gabi used to make a few repeat dishes that were always family favorites. This was when I first discovered I loved the smoky flavor of cumin. Her version of this soup offered an aroma in her kitchen that was so inviting. Cumin is a dynamic super spice that gives any dish a depth of flavor with a warming after-effect.

4 cups chicken broth, bone broth or vegetable stock

1 pound chicken breast

1 medium yellow or Spanish onion, chopped

2 garlic cloves, chopped or minced

1 yellow bell pepper, chopped

2 teaspoons ground cumin

1 teaspoon dried oregano

½ teaspoon chili powder

1 *(15-ounce)* can organic white northern or cannellini beans, drained and rinsed

2 tablespoons chopped fresh cilantro

1 *(4-ounce)* can diced green chilis

Sea salt and black pepper, to taste

In a large soup pot, add the broth and chicken, cover and cook over medium heat for about 15 minutes. Once the chicken is no longer pink, remove it from the pot and place it in a large bowl.

Add the chopped onion, garlic, and bell pepper to the pot and allow them to cook with the cover on while you shred the chicken with two forks. Return the shredded chicken to the pot and add the cumin, oregano, chili powder, beans, cilantro, and green chilis. Add salt and pepper to taste and stir until all ingredients are well combined.

Allow it to simmer for at least 15 minutes so all the flavors have a chance to party together.

Serve with diced avocado and watch the healthy goodness disappear from your bowl like magic.

Deliciously Holistic: Inspired Favorites

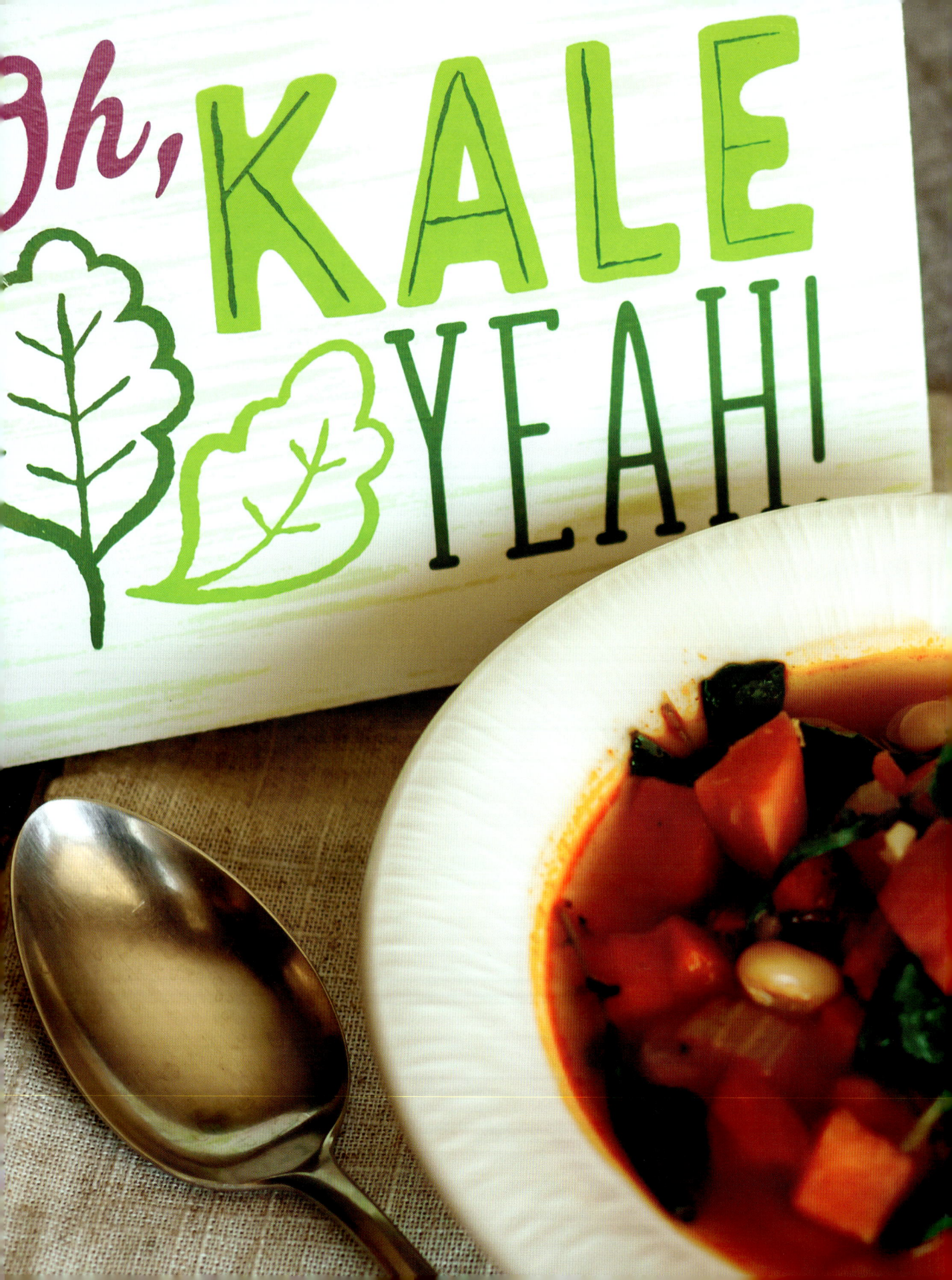

Smoky Sweet Potato Chowder

Although I support the benefits of and often promote the plant-based movement, I'm certainly no vegan. Let's take a moment to notice that I used two different terms here: vegan and plant-based. Vegans are very careful not to eat or use any item derived from animals. The strictest vegans don't even use typical lip balm due to it containing beeswax. Plant-based, however, focuses on meals consisting of plants; not a product that once was a plant, manipulated in a lab and then marketed as "meatless." Quite often my recipes come out of a simple craving for color, flavor and a comforting spoonful of goodness. When that happens, they are often organically meatless, and yet I love them just the same.

1 tablespoon coconut or avocado oil

1 medium yellow onion, chopped

2 medium celery stalks, chopped

2 medium carrots, chopped

1 bell pepper, chopped

2 cloves garlic, minced

Sea salt and black pepper, to taste

2 pounds sweet potatoes (*2 to 3 medium potatoes*), **peeled and diced**

1 teaspoon dried thyme

1 teaspoon smoked paprika

½ teaspoon ground sage

1 (*15-ounce*) **can organic white cannellini beans**

4 cups vegetable broth

4–5 cups baby kale

Heat the oil in a soup pot over medium heat. Add the onion, celery, carrots, and bell pepper and cook until the vegetables are soft and tender, about 6 to 8 minutes. Stir in the garlic and some sea salt and black pepper and cook for 1 minute. Add the sweet potatoes, thyme, paprika, sage, and beans and stir to combine and cook for 1 minute.

Add the broth and bring to a boil. Reduce the heat to maintain a simmer, cover and cook until the sweet potatoes are tender, 10 to 15 minutes.

Stir in the baby kale and allow it to wilt before serving.

After a bowl of this satisfying soup you may just look at plant-based cuisine with a little more lust. Go ahead and crave real food—I dare ya!

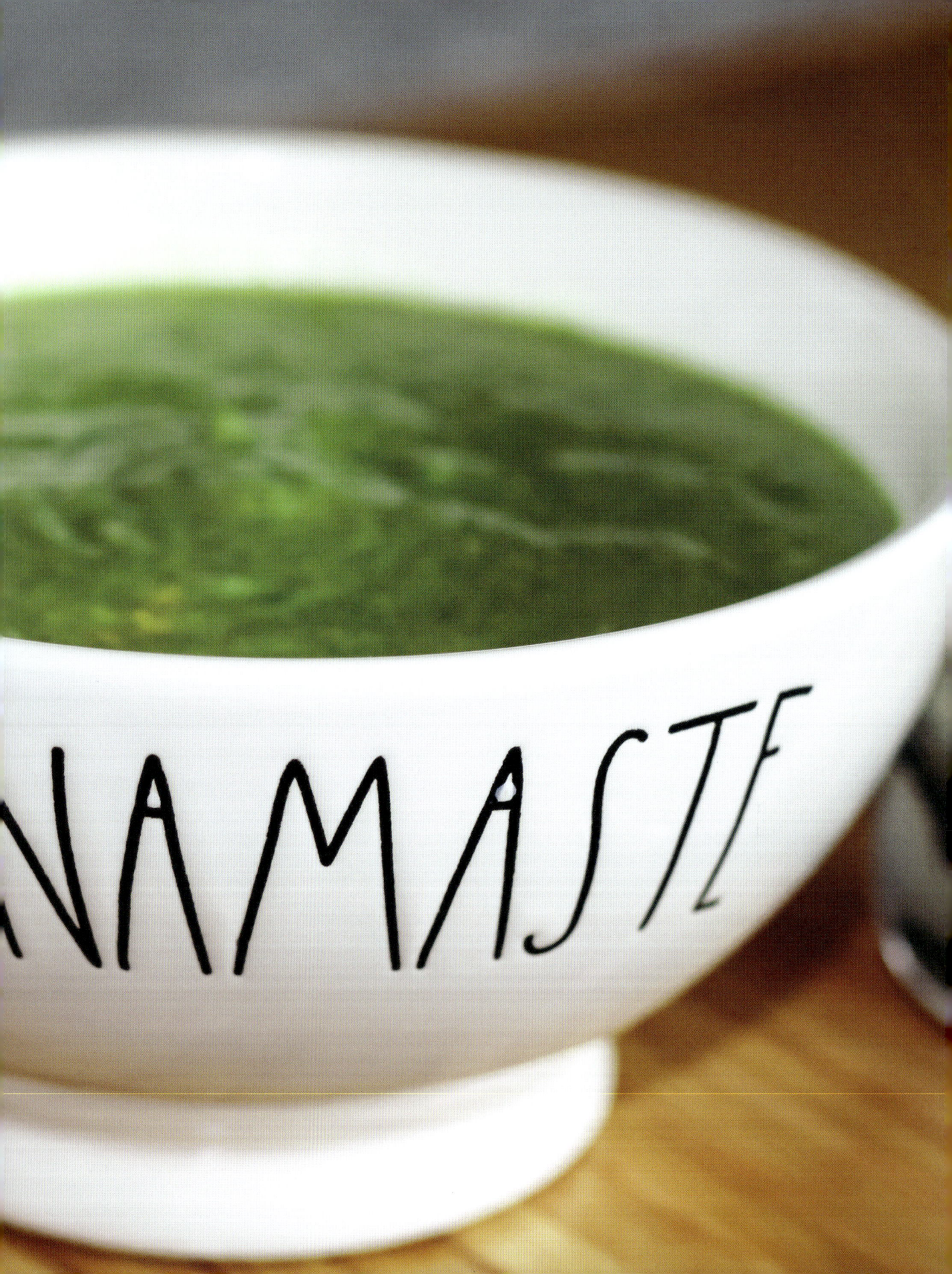

Supremely Delicious Broccoli Soup

My mother used to make a very thin, but lovely cream of broccoli soup that was just delish! As most of my mom's recipes of the past, it contained hefty amounts of half & half and margarine. I was determined to recreate this recipe and make it an incredible superfood soup—as it should be! Every ingredient in this version is packed with powerful, disease fighting properties and yes, just like mom's—it's delish!

- 1 tablespoon coconut oil
- 1 medium Spanish or yellow onion, chopped
- 2–3 celery stalks, chopped
- 8 oz of Portabella or cremini mushroom, chopped
- 2 garlic cloves, chopped
- Sea salt and black pepper, to taste
- 4 cups vegetable, bone or organic chicken broth
- 6 cups fresh broccoli florets
- 1 tablespoon fresh basil
- 1 tablespoon fresh parsley
- 1 *(15-ounce)* can organic white beans, drained and rinsed *(cannellini or white northern)*
- ¼ cup nutritional yeast
- Juice from ½ lemon

Heat coconut oil in a soup pot over medium heat. Add onion, celery and mushroom to the pot and sauté for 10–12 minutes until veggies begin to look soft. Stir in the garlic, season with salt and pepper and cook for 1 more minute. Next add broth, broccoli, basil, parsley and white beans, give it all a good stir and cover. Cook for another 10–12 minutes to allow the broccoli to cook.

Using an immersion blender, blend the soup to a creamy consistency. If you do not have an immersion blender, simply blend the soup in batches using your kitchen blender and add it back to the pot. Stir in nutritional yeast and fresh lemon juice.

Serve as an appetizer or as a lovely lunch and enjoy the delicious benefit of your time well spent.

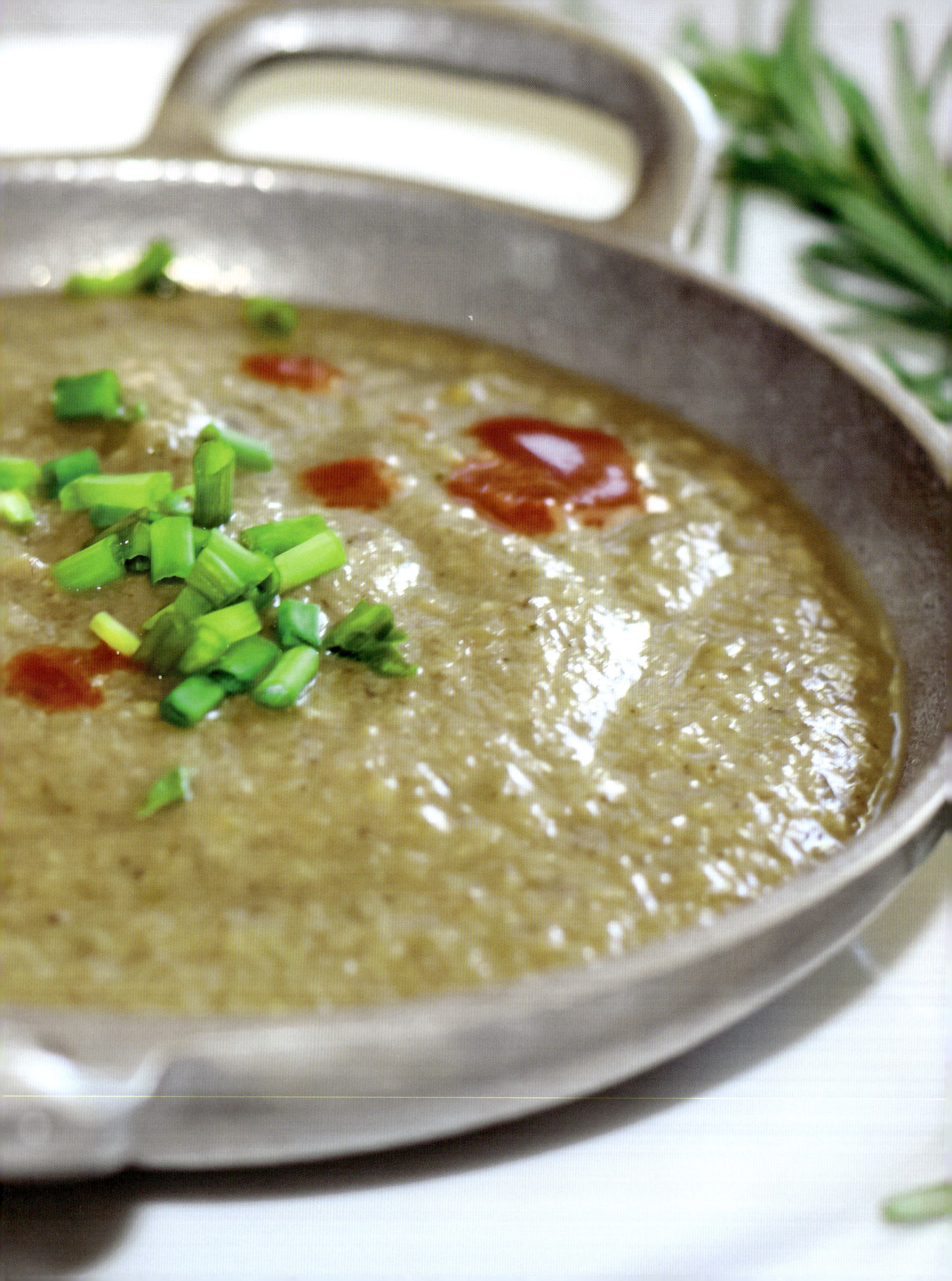

Mighty Mushroom Bisque

Mushrooms are an interesting food; some people love them, some people hate them and others learn to love them—like me! There are many types of mushrooms; some are edible and some are not. Some are used for medicinal purposes or to mimic meat in vegan dishes. I have learned to love them for the presence of Vitamin D as that is tough to obtain anywhere else in the produce aisle. I hope this soup inspires you to try to enjoy the mighty mushroom and its many uses in your kitchen.

1 tablespoon coconut oil

2 pounds of any blend of mushrooms such as shitake, maitake, oyster, crimini, Portabella, or any edible mushrooms you can get your hands on, roughly chopped

1 onion, chopped

1 yellow bell pepper, chopped

2 celery stalks, chopped

Sea salt and black pepper, to taste

3 garlic cloves, chopped

1 tablespoon fresh rosemary

2 teaspoons dried thyme

1 (15-ounce) can of organic white beans (cannellini or white northern)

3 cups vegetable or bone broth

¼ cup nutritional yeast (optional)

In a large soup pot, melt coconut oil over medium heat. Add chopped mushrooms, onion, bell pepper and celery to the pot. Cook veggies about 10 minutes or until the mushrooms begin to let off their juices and everything is looking soft. Season with sea salt and black pepper, and stir well. Add chopped garlic and allow to cook for one minute. Add chopped rosemary, thyme, and white beans and stir once again. Add broth, cover, reduce heat to medium low and simmer for 10 minutes, allowing for all the flavors to marry together.

Using an immersion blender, blend the soup until it is smooth and has a creamy consistency. If you do not own what is currently my favorite kitchen tool, simply ladle the soup into a blender in batches to create a smooth consistency. It's a bisque after all. Stir in the nutritional yeast and garnish with a dash of hot sauce and chopped green onion or fresh chives.

Serve confidently to anyone who claims to NOT enjoy mushrooms.

Tip: Don't run your mushrooms under water in attempt to clean them. They are little sponges after all and will absorb the water and add too much liquid to your soup. Simply wipe them with a damp cloth or paper towel to remove any residual dirt. If you are lucky enough to grow your own mushrooms in organic soil—a little dirt is actually good for you!

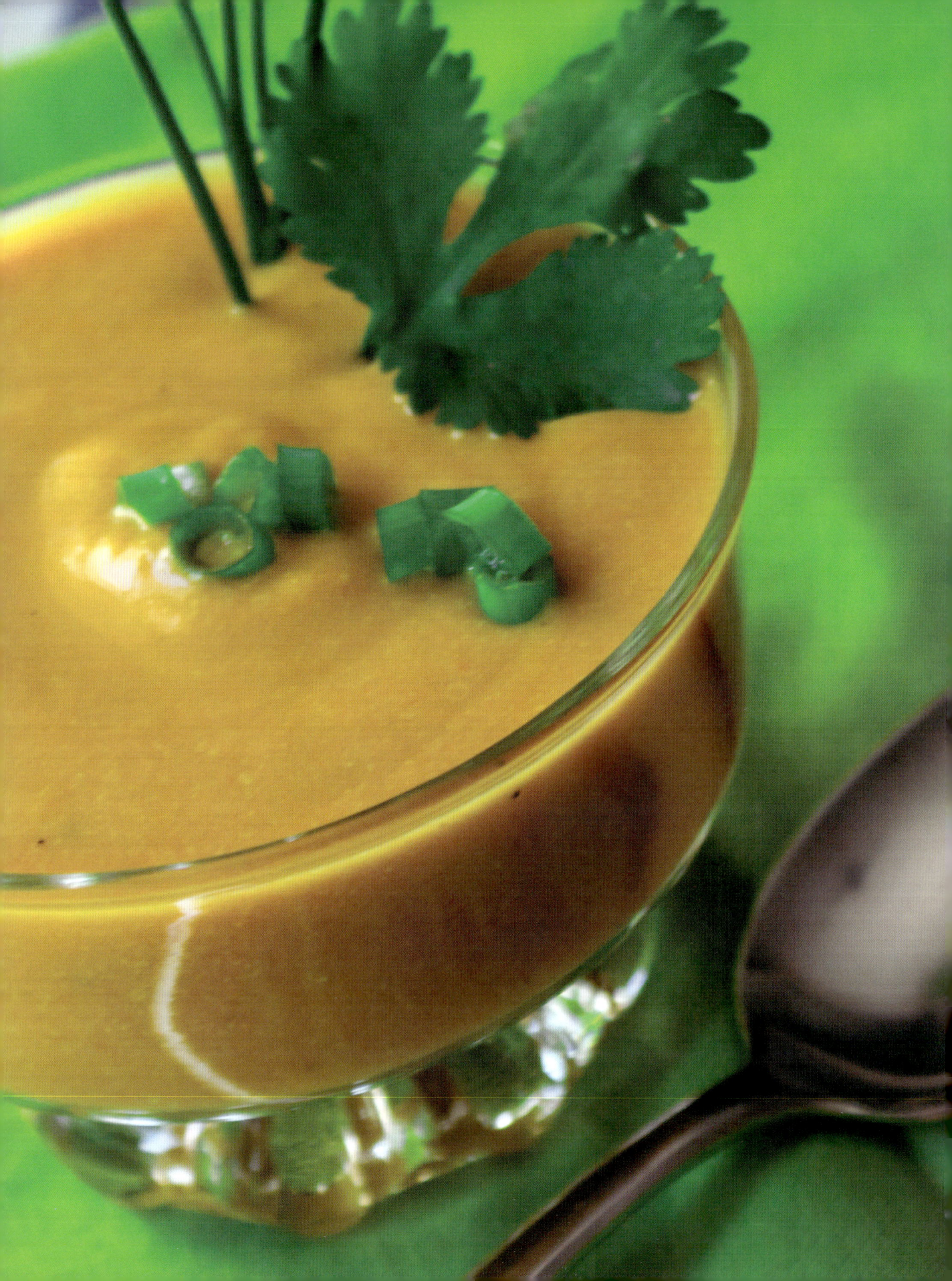

Gorgeous Ginger Cashew Carrot Soup

You have heard me say it before, and I will say again: Eat for color! As a general rule, the richer the color, the better a food is for you. This soup earned the title of gorgeous not only because of its radiant hue, but because of how its ingredients work together to make you feel truly gorgeous inside and out. I recommend you make this at least once a month to remind yourself of how the beauty of the Earth is meant for us to take in both in physical form and in a spiritual sense. I find it utterly impossible to consume a gorgeous meal such as this one and not appreciate how beautiful the world around us can be.

1 cup raw cashews, soaked and drained

6 carrots, peeled and chopped into 1-inch pieces

1 yellow onion, sliced

3 celery stalks, chopped into 1-inch pieces

1-inch piece of fresh ginger root, peeled

1 garlic clove, sliced

¼ teaspoon ground turmeric (you can certainly buy fresh turmeric root if it's available)

Sea salt and black pepper, to taste

4 cups vegetable broth

Chopped cilantro, green onion or chives as an optional garnish

Add cashews to a bowl and cover with water. Allow them to soak for a minimum of 1 hour as they will need to become very soft. Drain the liquid and set aside.

In a large soup pot, add the carrots, onion, celery, ginger, garlic, turmeric, sea salt, black pepper and vegetable broth and bring to a boil. Lower the heat to simmer, cover and cook for 20 minutes or until the carrots are fork tender.

Add the cashews and purée the soup using an immersion blender. If you do not have an immersion blender, simply transfer the soup in batches to a blender and return to the pot. Ladle a generous portion into your favorite bowl or mug and top with chopped cilantro, green onion or chives.

Since the preparation of this soup is simplified even more the others in this book, I ask that you use that extra time to think of a few other ways you can connect with nature throughout the week. Some of my personal favorites include getting my hands in the dirt, my feet in the grass, and when I am overly blessed, making a snow angel out of warm sand.

Deliciously Holistic: Inspired Favorites

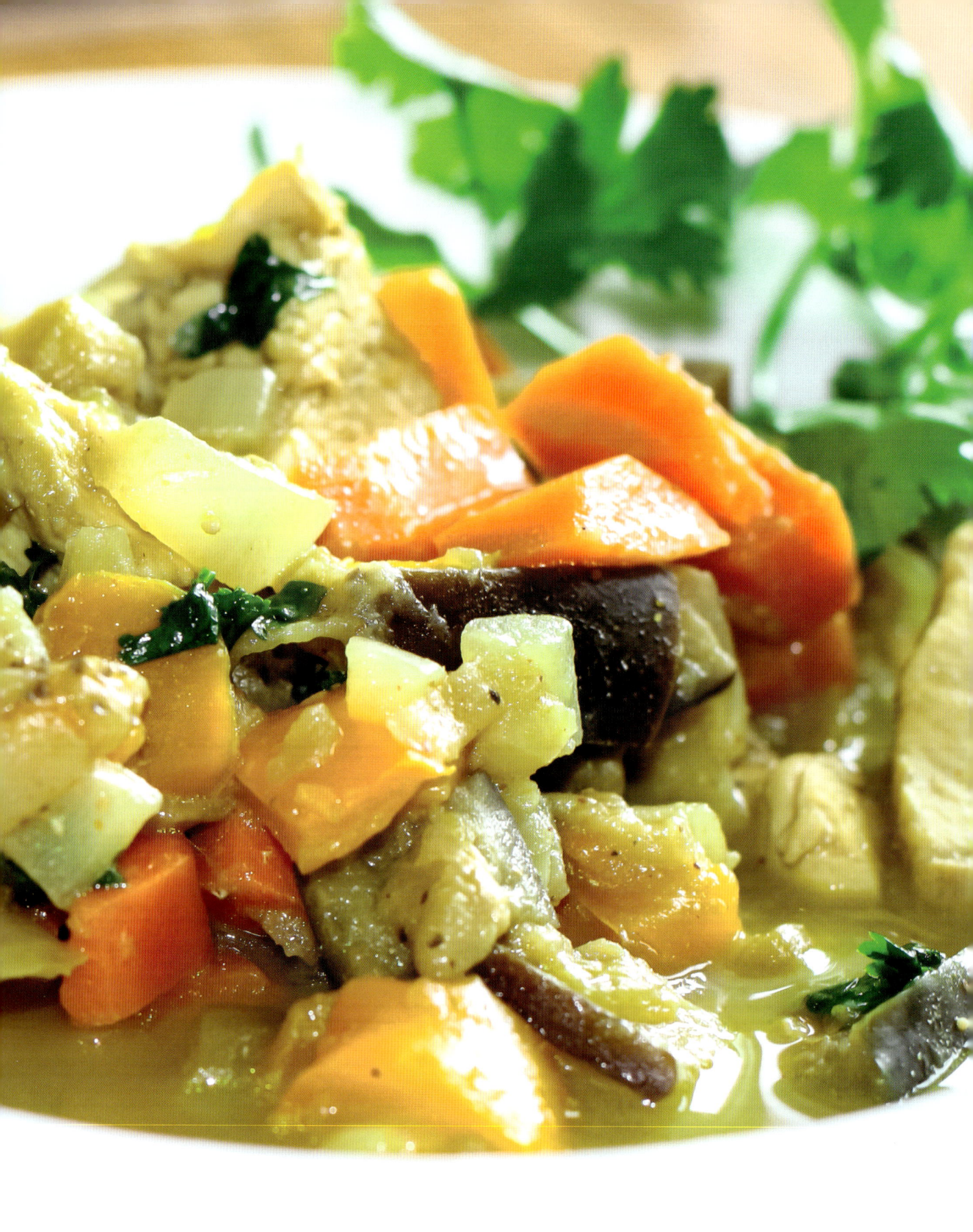

Comforting Curry Stew

You may think curry is one of those flavors that you either like or you don't. I would say that if you have already placed yourself in the don't category—give it another shot. Curry is actually a blend of spices as well as a style of cooking. As soon as the temperatures begin to drop, I start craving those warming flavors of cumin, ginger, and coriander; all of which are classic curry ingredients. Although the seasoning blend will vary based on the region it is created in or inspired by, you will certainly always end up with a flavorful, anti-inflammatory, delightful dish.

1 tablespoon coconut oil

1 medium yellow onion, chopped

1 orange bell pepper, chopped

2 medium carrots, chopped

1 medium eggplant, chopped

2 garlic cloves, finely chopped

Sea salt and black pepper, to taste

1 pound organic chicken breast, chopped into bite sized pieces

1 (*4-ounce*) can organic green chilis

1 teaspoon curry powder

2 cups chicken or vegetable broth

½ cup coconut milk

1 tablespoon almond or cashew butter *(make sure to buy a brand with no sugar added)*

½ cup fresh cilantro leaves

In a large soup pot, heat coconut oil over medium heat. Add onion, bell pepper, carrots and eggplant and sauté for 8–10 minutes until the veggies get soft. Add the garlic and some sea salt and black pepper and cook for one minute more.

Add the chunks of chicken breast and cook until no longer pink on the outside, stirring occasionally. Next stir in the green chilis and curry powder until everything is well coated in the pot. Add the broth, cover the pot, and allow to simmer for 8–10 minutes.

In a small bowl, combine the coconut milk with the almond butter and blend into the stew. Top with fresh cilantro and enjoy the comforting warmth of a nutritiously crafted stew.

Tip: To make this a delicious vegan dish, simply swap out the chicken for a 15-ounce can of organic chickpeas.

Deliciously Holistic: Inspired Favorites

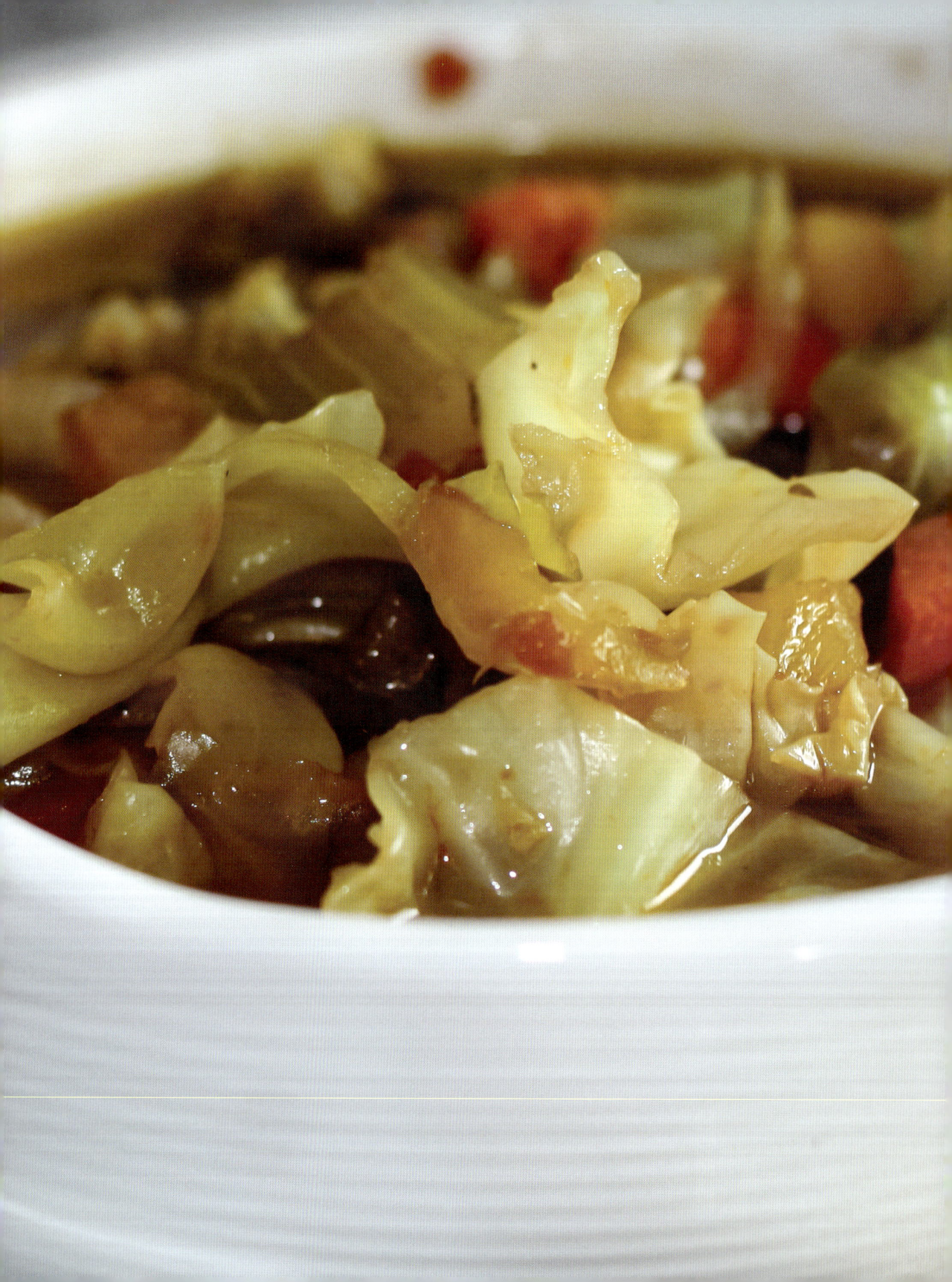

Cleverly Sweetened Cabbage Soup

The first time I enjoyed this soup, I was a young gal still confused about what was healthy and what was not. I was so proud of myself for enjoying multiple bowls as I had agreed to try it simply because I believed I was making an obvious healthy choice. Then I went searching for a recipe to make in my own little apartment kitchen. It wasn't long before I discovered the secret ingredient to this popular, diet trendy food: BROWN SUGAR. Don't be confused; that is just white sugar mixed with molasses. And no, it is not good for you. But this recipe, like all others, deserves to be as nutritious as it is delicious. Holistic Health by Valerie to the rescue. I'll bet after you make this for yourself, you will also discover why this version is surprisingly sweet (without the deception, of course).

1 tablespoon coconut oil

1 yellow or Spanish onion, chopped

1 yellow bell pepper, chopped

2 medium carrots, chopped into bite sized pieces

2–3 celery stalks, chopped

2 garlic cloves, chopped

Sea salt and black pepper, to taste

1 (15-ounce) can organic chopped tomatoes

⅓ cup balsamic vinegar

⅛ teaspoon crushed red pepper flakes

1 medium-sized head green cabbage, thinly sliced

8 cups vegetable broth

In a large soup pot, melt coconut oil over medium heat and add the onion, bell pepper, carrot and celery. Cook for about 5-7 minutes until the veggies start to look soft, stirring occasionally. Stir in the garlic, salt and pepper and cook for 1 minute. Next, add the tomatoes, balsamic vinegar, crushed red pepper and cabbage.

Stir well to combine all ingredients. Add vegetable broth and bring the temperature up until you achieve a low boil. Cover the pot, bring temperature down to medium low and simmer for 30 minutes. Give it a taste test and add a touch more sea salt, black pepper or crushed red pepper if necessary.

Enjoy this soup on a day you feel you are needing to recharge, reset or rebalance. You can also make in advance, freeze, and have on hand when the same need arises with no time to spare.

Dee-Lish Dinners

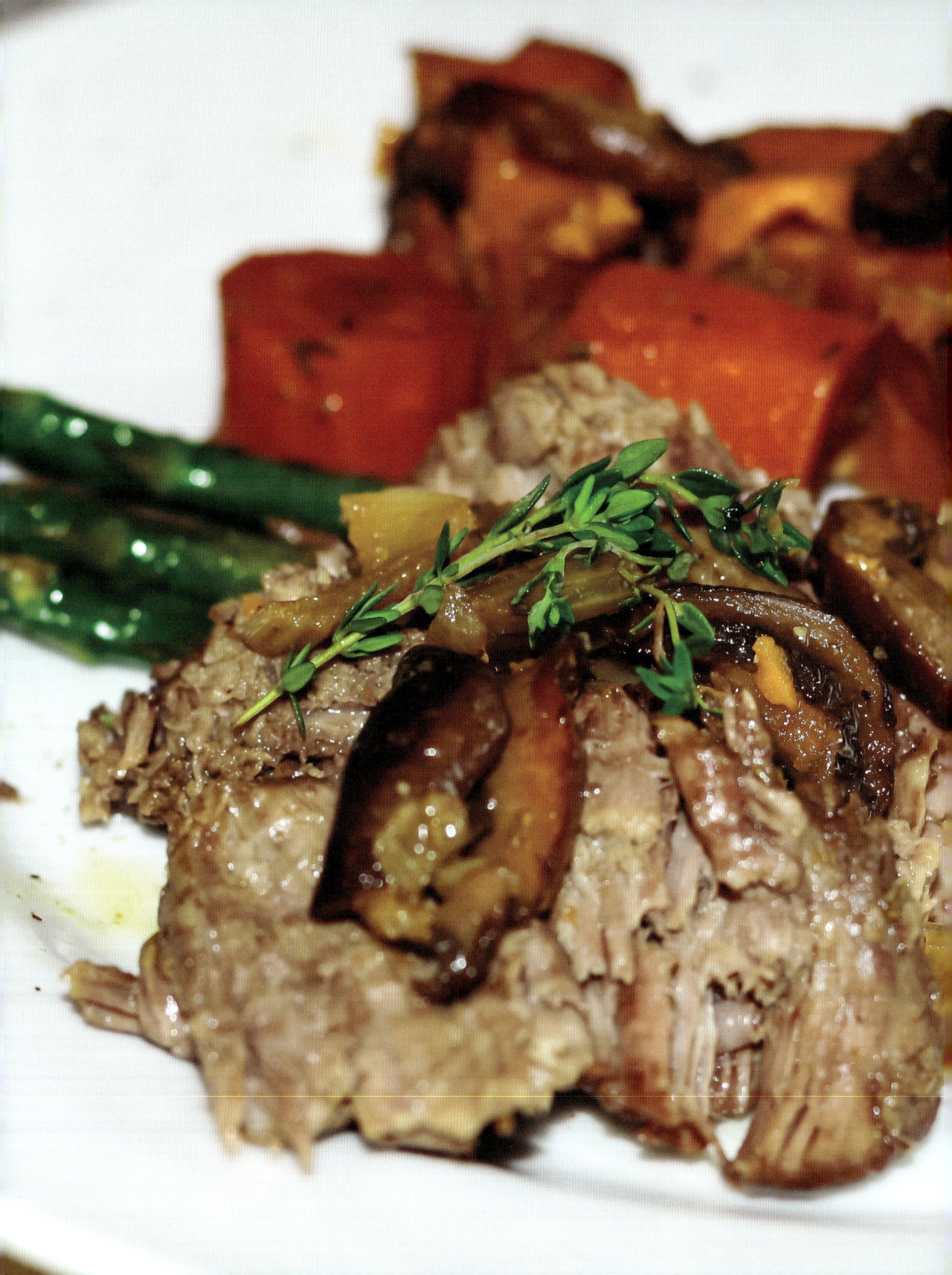

Please Eat Pot Roast

In case you were still confused, red meat is not the enemy. Simply the way we eat red meat is the problem. The majority of our cows are being fed genetically modified grains when they should be eating grass. We also eat exceptionally large portions and processed versions of what was once beef. Buy an organic, grass-fed roast from a reputable source, fill your plate ¾ of the way full with colorful veggies and savor every bite.

24 oz. chuck or shoulder roast

Sea salt and black pepper, to taste

1 tablespoon coconut oil

1 medium onion, chopped

4 celery stalks, chopped

8 ounces mushrooms, sliced *(optional)*

2 cloves garlic, finely chopped

1 tablespoon fresh thyme leaves *(or 1 teaspoon dried)*

1 tablespoon fresh rosemary *(or 1 teaspoon dried)*

2 cups organic beef broth *(beef bone broth is best)*

2–3 medium sweet potatoes, unpeeled and chopped into approximately 2-inch chunks

4–6 medium sized carrots, peeled and chopped into approximately 1-inch chunks

Share this meal with anyone worthy of a hug at the end of the day.

Carefully trim any excess fat without disrupting the integrity of the roast. Pat the roast with paper towel and season each side with sea salt and black pepper. Heat 1 tablespoon of coconut oil in a large Dutch oven over medium heat. Add the meat and brown for 3–5 minutes on each side. Remove from the pot and set aside.

Add onion, celery and mushrooms *(if using)* and continue cooking for about 5–6 minutes, stirring occasionally. Stir in the garlic, thyme and rosemary and allow to cook for one minute more. Add broth and stir well, scraping up all of the brown bits *(aka the flavor)* stuck to the bottom of the pot. Turn off the heat. Return the roast to the pot, and add the sweet potatoes and carrots by arranging them around and on top of the meat. Cover with the lid and cook for 2 hours in a 325-degree oven.

Don't have two hours to stay home with your oven on? No problem! For a slow cooker option, follow instructions above but instead of using a Dutch oven, simply use a large enough pan *(I prefer cast iron)* to sear your meat and cook your veggies and herbs. Once you "turn off the heat," transfer the entire contents of the pan to the slow cooker, add the beef on top and then the carrots and sweet potatoes. Cook on low for 6 hours. Now you are free to go about your day and will return home to an incredible aroma coming from your kitchen. Love—it is the smell of pure love in a pot.

Deliciously Holistic: Inspired Favorites

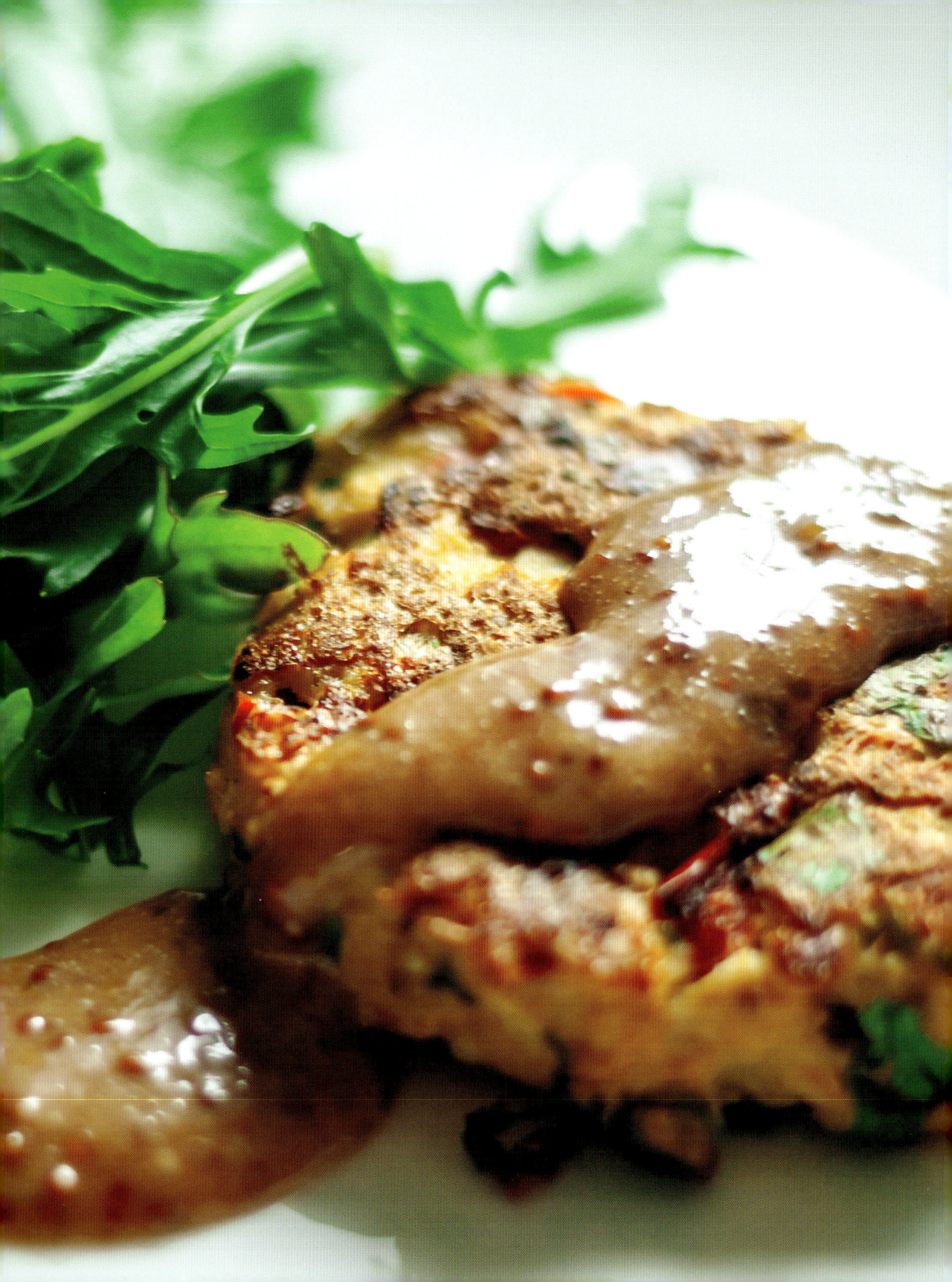

No Reason to be Crabby with these Crab Cakes

Sometimes life will give you lemons. A day, a week, or even a season can sometimes just seem to be bringing you down. When I find myself feeling crabby over life's lemons, I lift myself up with a decadent dinner that's reserved for special occasions. What's so special about today? You are! Treat yourself to this delightful meal and know that something great is just around the corner. Until then, at least something delicious is soon to be on your plate.

1 egg

8 ounces wild-caught white crab meat, drained

½ cup red bell pepper, petite diced

¼ cup fresh cilantro, chopped

¼ cup green onion, chopped

1 tablespoon hemp seed

1 tablespoon nutritional yeast

1 teaspoon Cajun seasoning

1 teaspoon ground mustard

Sea salt and black pepper, to taste

1 teaspoon coconut or avocado oil

Plenty of arugula

1 lemon, cut into wedges

Drizzling sauce

1 tablespoon whole grain mustard

1 tablespoon avocado oil mayo

2 tablespoons raspberry, cherry or plum preserves or jam with no added sugar

In a medium bowl, crack one egg and whisk it with a fork to break up the yolk. Add the crab, bell pepper, cilantro, green onion, hemp seed, nutritional yeast, Cajun seasoning, mustard and some sea salt and black pepper. Using your hand, combine all ingredients and shape the mixture into four individual patties and set aside.

Melt oil in a large skillet over medium heat. Add the crab cakes to the hot pan and cook for 7–9 minutes on each side.

Whisk sauce ingredients together in a bowl until well combined.

Pile a good amount of arugula on your plate. Add 1–2 crab cakes on the greens and drizzle the sauce over each cake. Squeeze a few lemon wedges over the top and enjoy!

Life will always give us a lemon now or then, just be sure to use it as nature intended—with homemade crab cakes.

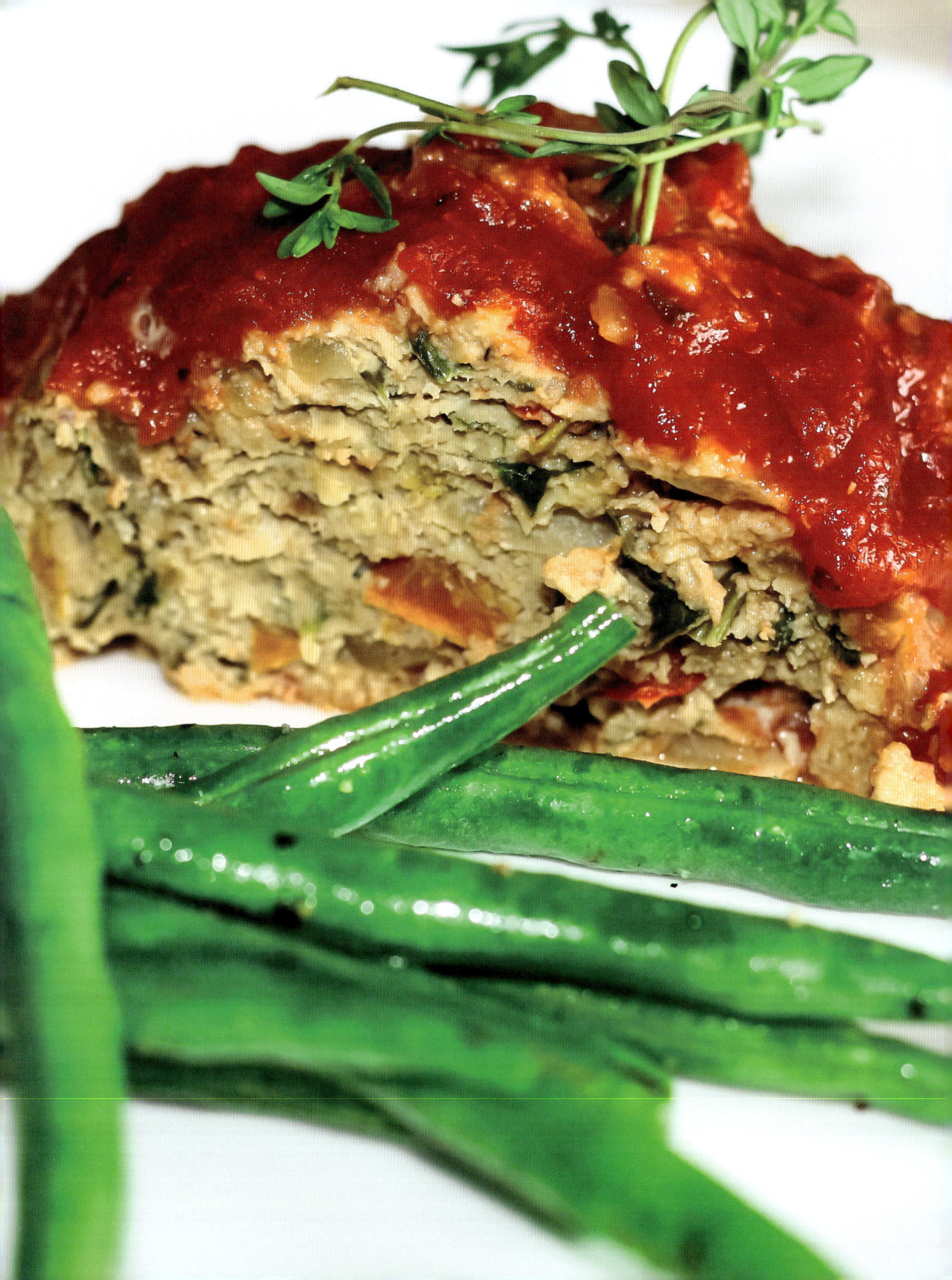

Truly Tasty Turkey Meatloaf

For decades, experts have asked us to replace our beloved beef for a turkey alternative. I understand this is not always a welcomed swap as I too have suffered restaurant remorse after ordering what proved to be a dry and tasteless turkey burger. Fear not! This recipe will leave you wondering how turkey can be so flavorful and satisfying without the cranberries and stuffing.

- 1 ¼ cups good quality marinara *(ensure there is NO added sugar)*
- 1 teaspoon coconut or avocado oil
- 1 small onion, petite diced
- 1 red bell pepper, petite diced
- 4 ounces mushrooms, thinly sliced
- 1 garlic clove, finely chopped
- 1 ½ teaspoons fresh thyme leaves
- 1 ½ teaspoons fresh oregano leaves
- Sea salt and black pepper, to taste
- 1 pound organic ground turkey
- 1 egg
- 1 cup fresh spinach, finely chopped
- 1 teaspoon balsamic vinegar
- ½ cup nutritional yeast
- ½ cup quick cooking oats

In a glass or ceramic baking dish, spread a thin layer of marinara along the bottom and set aside. In a medium skillet, heat oil over medium heat and add the onion, bell pepper and mushrooms. Sauté for about 8–10 minutes until the veggies get nice and soft.

Stir in the garlic, thyme, oregano and a little sea salt and black pepper and cook for 1 minute. Remove from the heat and allow to cool.

In a large bowl combine turkey, egg, spinach, balsamic vinegar, nutritional yeast, oats, veggie and herb mix and a little more sea salt and black pepper. Place mixture into the sauce lined baking dish and form into a loaf. Cover with the remaining sauce and cook uncovered in a preheated 375-degree oven for 45–50 minutes.

Serve with your favorite green vegetable and be sure to leave a portion for tomorrow's lunch. It just may be the highlight of your workday.

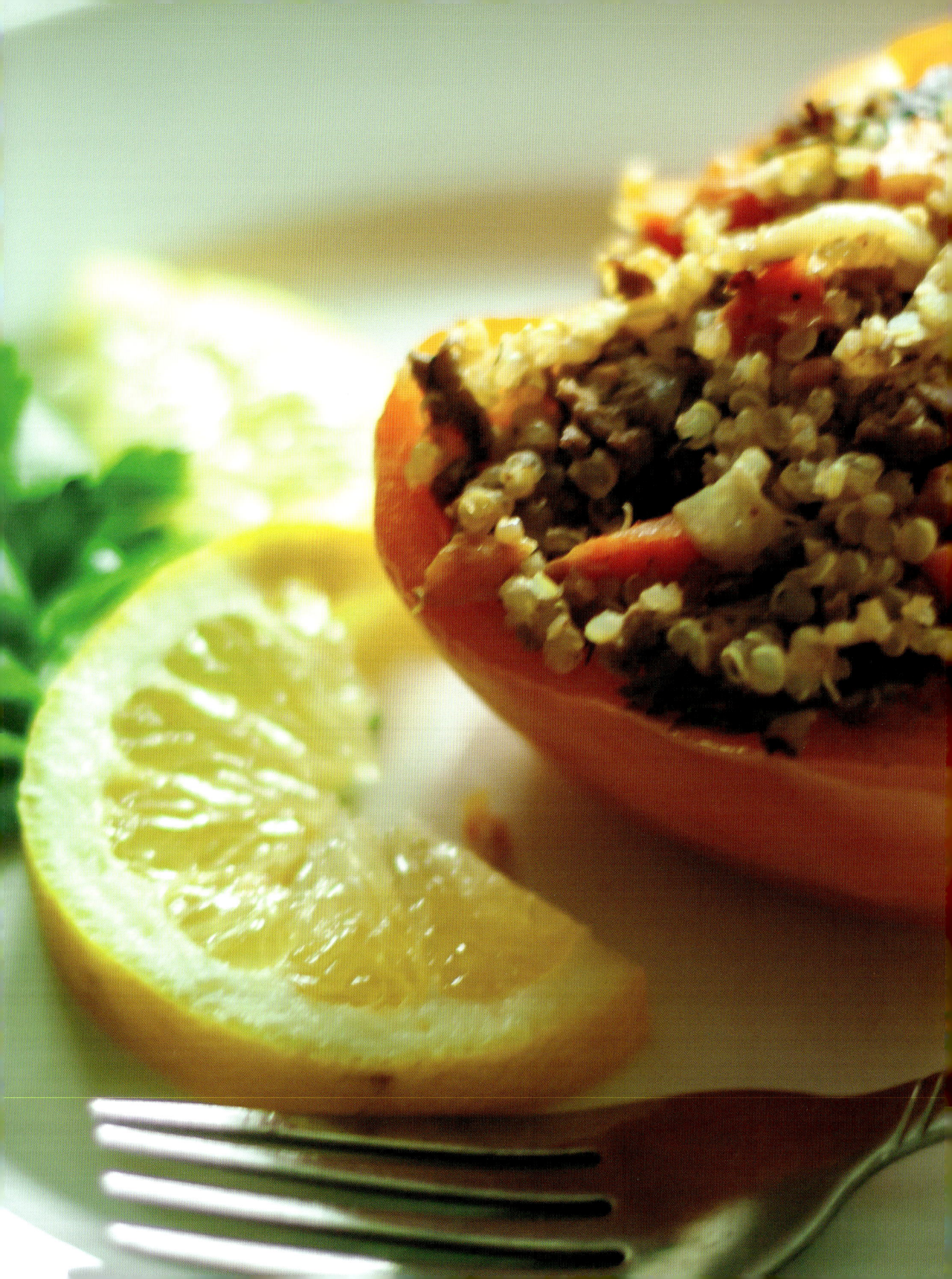

Summertime Stuffed Peppers

This recipe highlights everything great about summer: fresh herbs, juicy tomatoes and colorful bell peppers that are abundantly ripe for the picking. However, summer seems to fly by quicker than we would like, and I certainly don't want my readers feeling like they are stuck in their kitchen on a precious sunny day. If you are feeding an entire household of mouths, I recommend making a double batch, allowing this meal to be your lunch throughout the week. Ask a coworker to join you while you take your lunch break outdoors, or simply invite a neighbor to share the leftovers on your patio. Pair it with a mixed green salad full of cucumber and radish and enjoy a perfect celebration of summer's beauty.

1 teaspoon coconut oil

1 yellow onion, finely chopped

1 cup carrot, petite diced

1–2 garlic cloves, finely chopped

1 pound organic ground beef or lamb

Sea salt and black pepper to taste

2 cups Roma tomatoes, diced

1 cup fresh parsley, chopped

1 tablespoon fresh dill, chopped

Juice from ½ lemon

¼ cup nutritional yeast *(optional)*

1 cup cooked quinoa

4 bell peppers, cut in half lengthwise with the stem, ribs and seeds discarded

Preheat oven to 375 degrees.

In a large skillet, heat coconut oil over medium heat. Add onion and carrot and sauté for 4–6 minutes until the veggies begin to soften. Add the garlic, ground beef or lamb, and some sea salt and black pepper and cook until the meat is browned. Next stir in the tomatoes, parsley, dill, lemon juice and nutritional yeast *(if using)* and cook for 1–2 minutes. Finally add the quinoa and stir well to ensure all ingredients are thoroughly combined.

Place prepared peppers in a large baking dish with half an inch of water in the bottom. This will help to steam the peppers and prevent the bottoms from burning. Spoon the mixture into each pepper making sure they are well packed and filled to the top. Cover the pan and place in the oven for 45–50 minutes until the peppers are soft.

Remove from the oven, uncover and enjoy the incredible aroma. You think that part is great? Wait until you taste it.

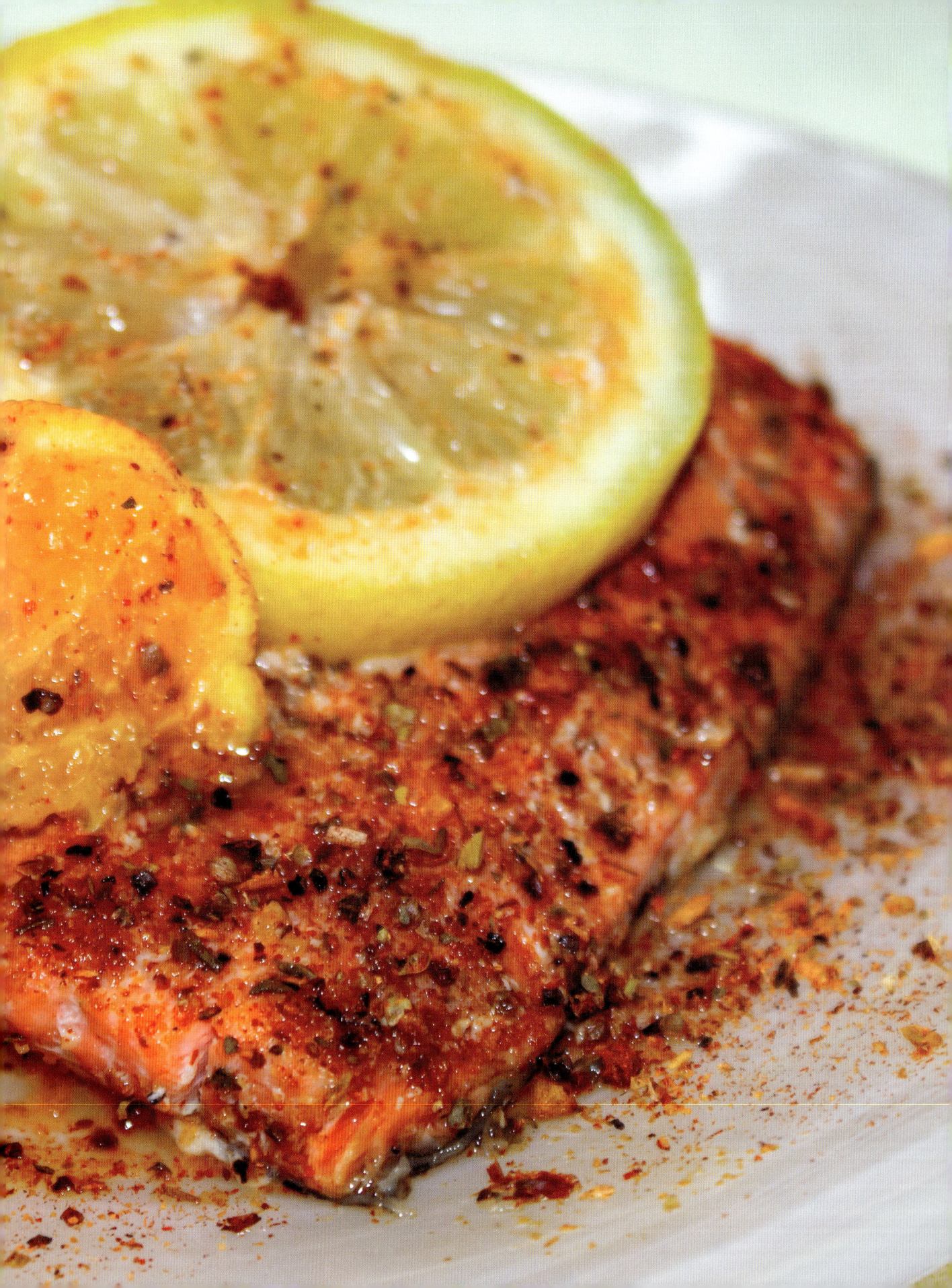

Simple Citrus Cajun Salmon

The best part of traveling is enjoying the local cuisine. Whenever we travel to seaside towns, I regularly seek out the small mom-and-pop restaurants with their own fishing boats. The absolute best meals come from those that feature a same-day-caught piece of fish with very few other ingredients. When your food is fresh and of the highest quality, you don't need much else but a little seasoning and some fresh citrus to bring out its beautiful flavor.

1 pound wild-caught salmon

Cajun or blackened seasoning

Lemon and orange slices

Preheat the oven to 375 degrees.

Line a glass or ceramic baking dish with enough parchment paper that it will double over the fish.

Pat the salmon with a paper towel and place skin side down in the pan. Sprinkle a generous amount of Cajun seasoning onto the salmon and gently pat it down without disturbing the flesh. Layer orange and lemon slices on the entire surface of the seasoned fish giving a mini squeeze to each piece as it goes down.

Bring the ends of the parchment paper together and fold over to create a little pouch for the fish to steam in.

Cook for 20 minutes or a little less if you prefer your salmon medium or medium well.

Serve with a large green salad and some homemade citrus iced tea. Add sunshine and enjoy.

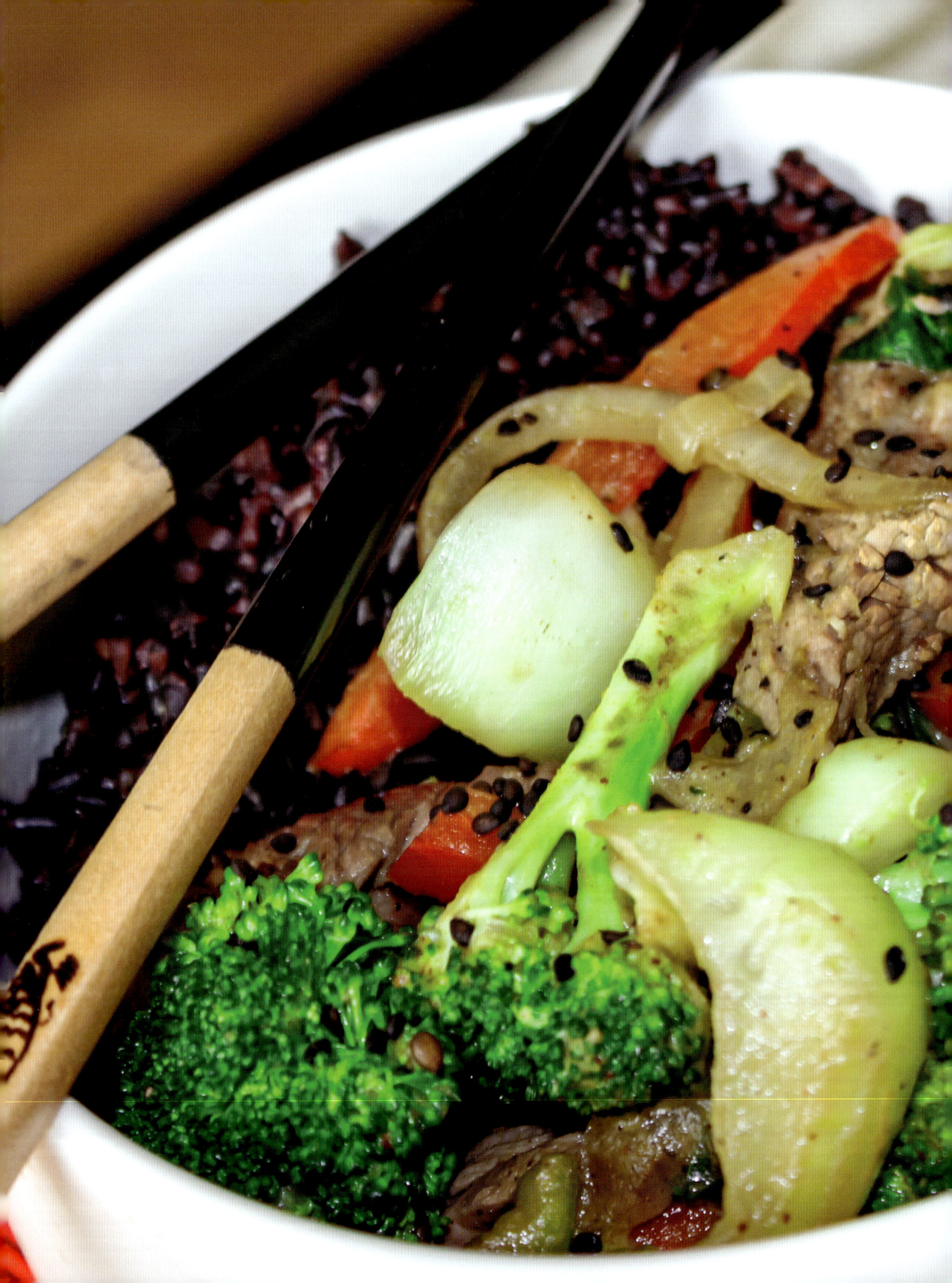

Curried Beef Stir Fry

Before this book was created, my recipes were reserved for clients and class guests only. Some recipes are designed for budding home cooks while others are meant for truly committed holistic all-stars. No matter where a person is on their wellness journey, one undeniable truth rings true: ultimately you need to chop some veggies, get them in a hot pan, and repeat regularly. Inspired by that philosophy, I created this recipe to give you all-star nutrition with fool-proof flavor.

1 ½ pound flank steak

Sea salt and black pepper, to taste

1 tablespoon green curry paste
(feel free to use red curry paste if you like more heat)

1 tablespoon almond butter

⅓ cup unsweetened coconut milk

1 tablespoon coconut oil

1 yellow onion, thinly sliced

1 red bell pepper, thinly sliced

2 cups broccoli, chopped

2 cups baby bok choy, chopped

1 tablespoon sesame seeds

Season both sides of the flank steak with sea salt and black pepper and set aside.

Combine curry paste, almond butter, and coconut milk in a bowl and set aside.

In a large wok or cast-iron skillet, add coconut oil and allow it to melt over medium-high heat. Add flank steak and sear for 2-3 minutes on each side. Remove steak from the skillet and place it on a cutting board. Add onion, bell pepper, broccoli, and bok choy to the skillet and keep the ingredients moving to avoid burning any of the veggies. Sauté for 3-5 minutes or until the veggies are cooked but not soft.

Pour the sauce mixture over the veggies and stir to combine. Turn down the heat slightly so your veggies do not get overcooked. Thinly slice the beef against the grain and add to the skillet along with the sesame seeds. You may need to move the beef around the pan until it is cooked to desired temperature.

Repeat regularly with or without the steak. Swap out different veggies as the seasons change and learn to use chopsticks. If nothing else it will force you to eat slower offering a few additional minutes to appreciate your culinary prowess.

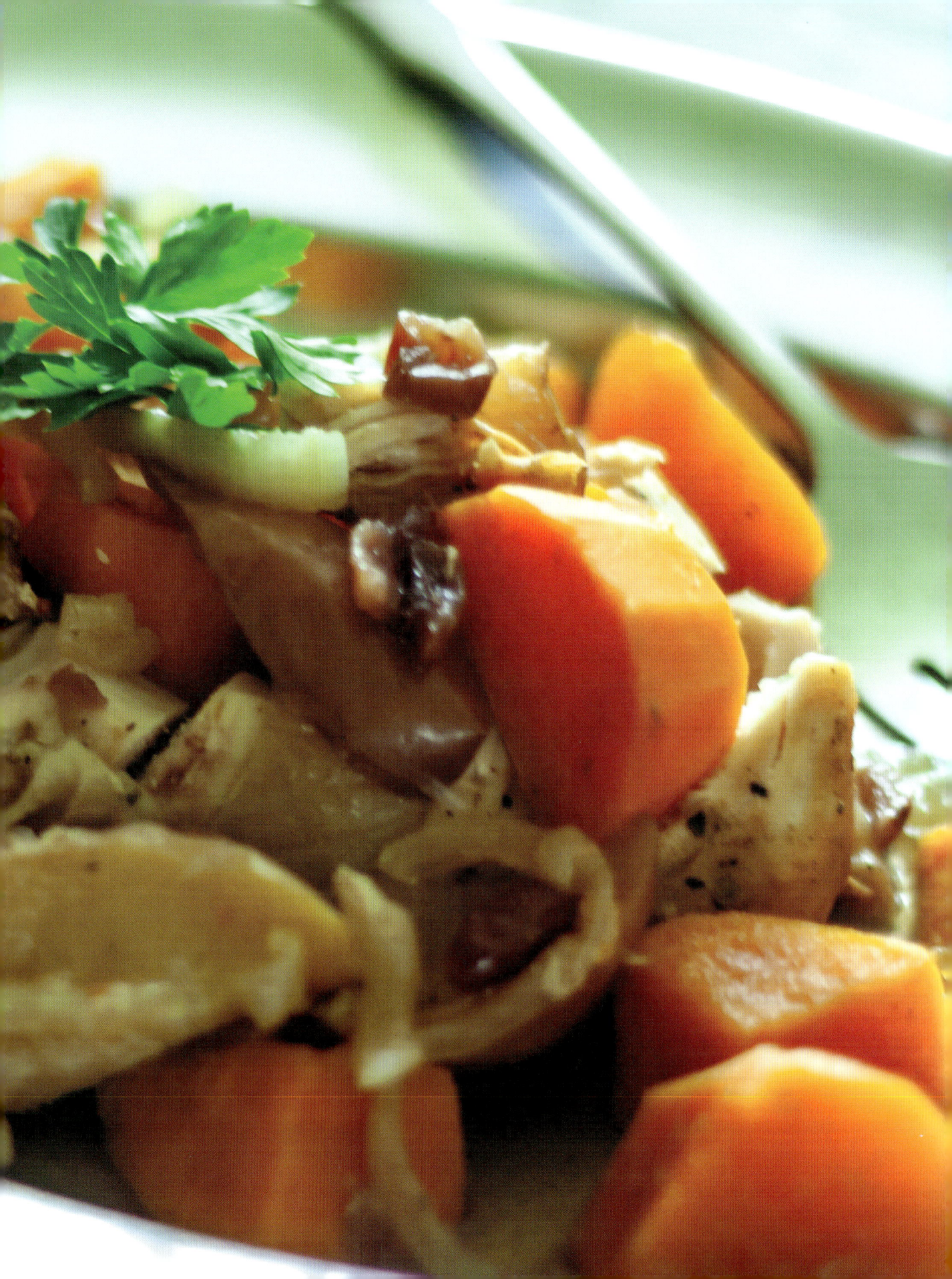

Thanksgiving on a Tuesday

Most holidays include a celebration of food. If you are like many Americans, you inevitably buy chocolate on Valentine's Day, barbeque on the 4th of July, and make cookies at Christmastime. But without question, the most anticipated meal of the year, and certainly the most palate pleasing holiday, is Thanksgiving. Whether you prepare it yourself, visit a friend or relative, or dine in a restaurant on this traditionally turkey-filled day, you will most likely encounter the same foods and flavors anywhere you go. This recipe offers you the perfect opportunity to enjoy Thanksgiving dinner any day of the year—even on a Tuesday.

1 ½–2 pound turkey tenderloin

1 medium onion, sliced

3 apples, cored and sliced

2 medium sweet potatoes, peeled and cut into 1-inch chunks

1 teaspoon dried sage

¼ teaspoon cardamom

¾ cup dried cranberries

1 cup vegetable broth

Sea salt and black pepper, to taste

Place the turkey tenderloin in the bottom of your slow cooker. In a large bowl, combine all other ingredients and pour the mixture over the turkey. Cover and cook on high for 4 hours or on low for up to 8 hours.

Remove the turkey, slice into thick pieces, and place on a serving platter. Portion some of the remaining ingredients along the top of the turkey and the rest along the sides. Skip the stuffing and enjoy with a little quinoa or sprouted wild rice.

Whether you are dining alone or enjoying this meal with loved ones, take a moment to acknowledge three things you are thankful for. My own moments of gratitude often include the Earth's beauty, the healing power of the human body, and avocados. (You didn't think I was going to forget about my favorite green food, did you?)

Deliciously Holistic: Inspired Favorites

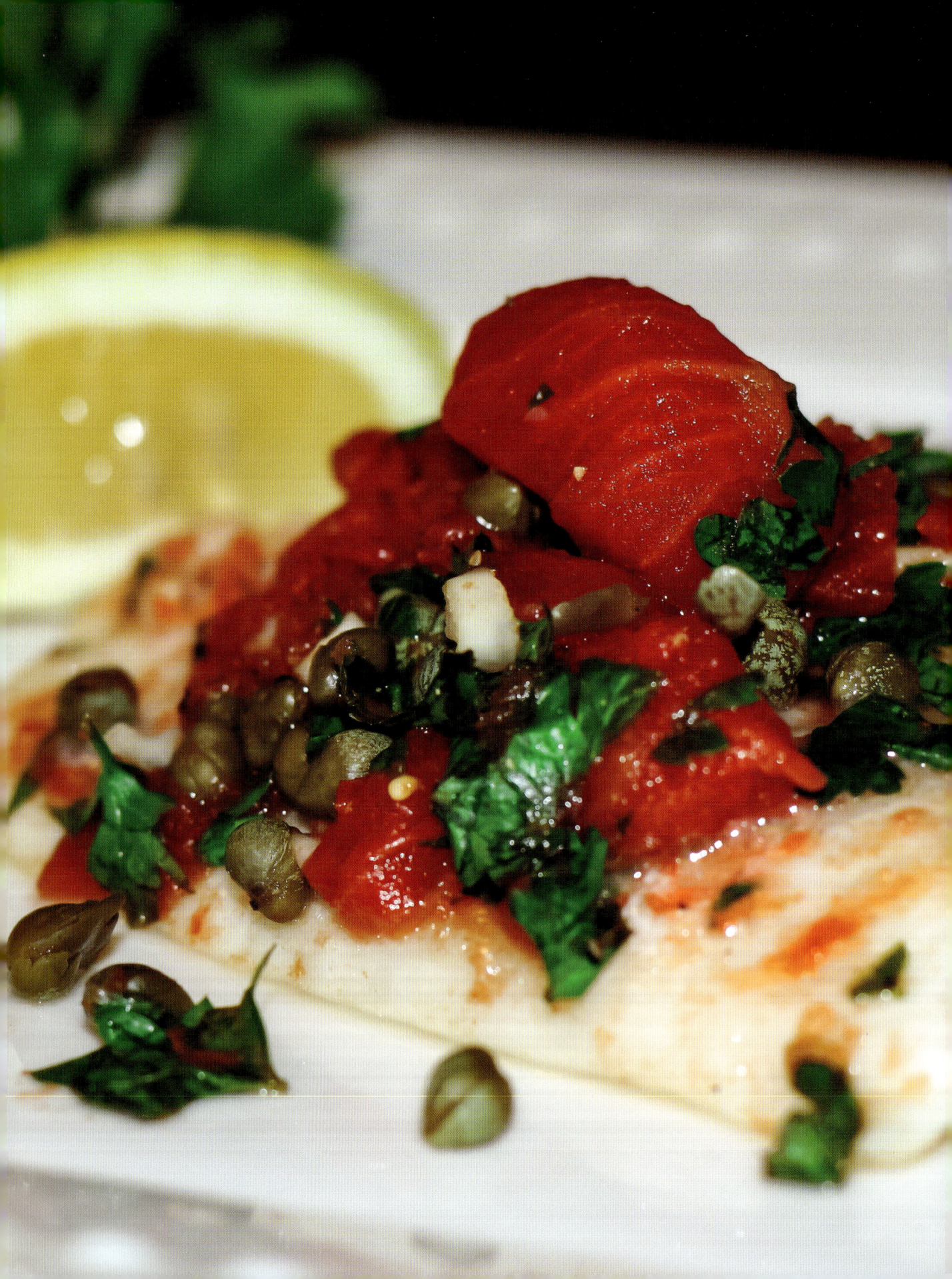

Taste of Venice Orange Roughy

Due to its placement on the sea, Venetian cuisine is known for its fresh fish and clean, bright flavors. Paired with fresh parsley and plenty of lemon, this dish is as simple as it is delicious. Even if you can't get to Venice for dinner tonight, you can certainly bring a little Venetian flair to your kitchen at home.

2 cups tomatoes, seeded & chopped

2 garlic cloves, finely chopped

½ cup fresh Italian parsley, chopped

¼ cup capers

Juice from 1 large lemon

Sea salt and black pepper, to taste

4 wild-caught orange roughy filets *(or any mild white fish)*

Preheat oven to 350 degrees.

In a medium-sized bowl, combine tomato, garlic, parsley, capers, lemon juice and some sea salt and freshly ground black pepper and set aside. Gently pat the fish with some paper towel to remove excess moisture and place side by side in a baking pan lined with parchment paper. Pour the tomato mixture on top of the fish, spreading it evenly over the 4 filets.

Place in the oven and cook for 15–20 minutes. Remove from the oven and serve immediately with a glass of chilled white wine.

Since preparing this dish took almost no time at all, take a few moments to sit, eat and enjoy conversation with loved ones. This is how it is done in Venice, after all.

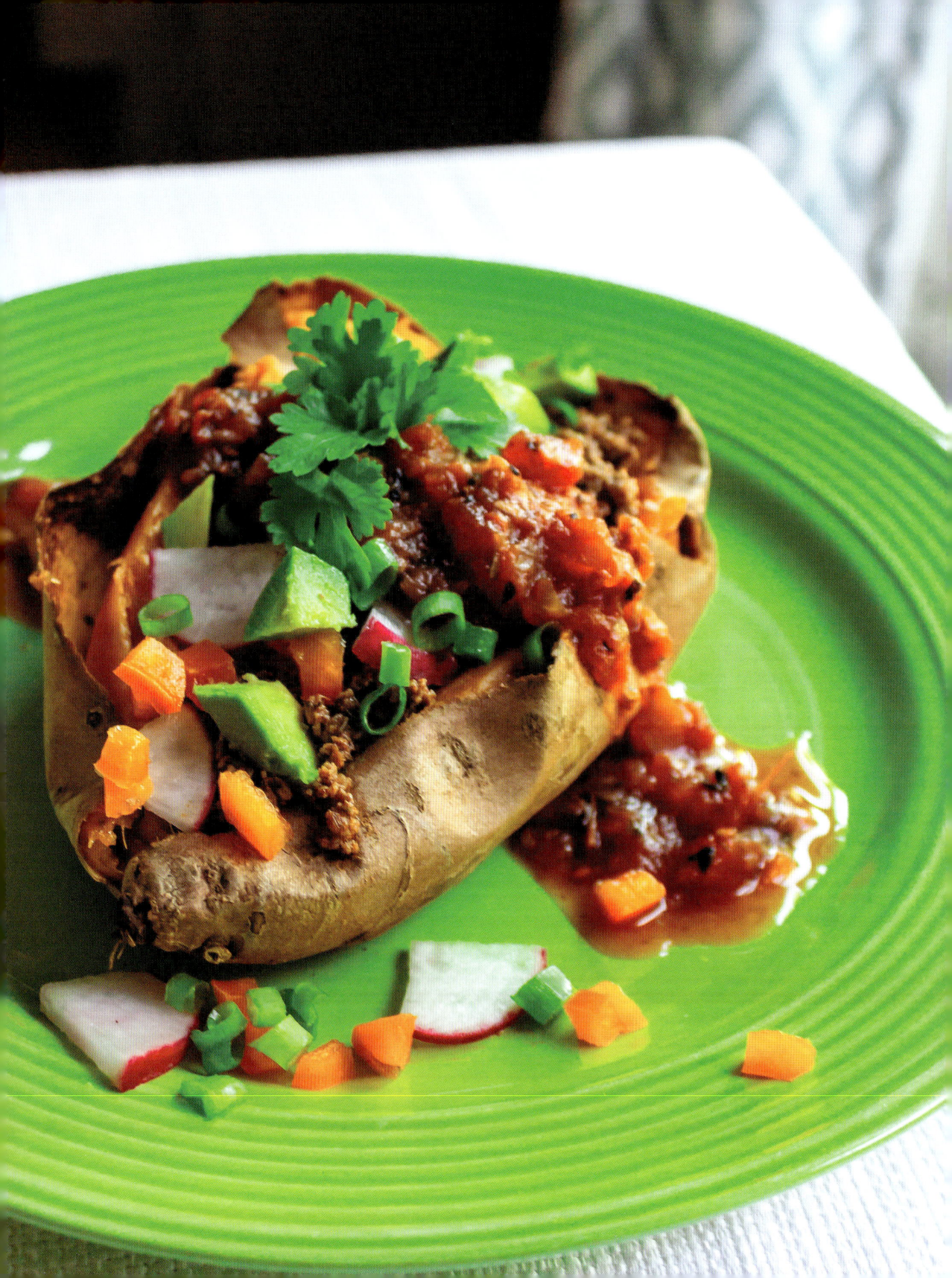

Sweet Po-Tacos

Who doesn't love a good taco night? The flavors are undeniable, but the ingredients can be questionable when it comes to nutrition. As you may have guessed, mine is free from shredded cheese, sour cream and yes—even the beloved corn shell. And yet, the biggest nutritional upgrade here is probably the seasoning. Typical taco seasoning packets can contain MSG (monosodium glutamate), artificial colors, and hydrogenated and hydrolyzed ingredients. No Bueno! This recipe will give you plenty of fiesta-style flavor without compromising the quality of ingredients.

4 medium sweet potatoes

1 teaspoon coconut oil

1 pound organic ground beef or ground turkey

1 (4-ounce) can diced green chilis

1 tablespoon chili powder

1 teaspoon dried oregano

1 teaspoon garlic powder

Sea salt and black pepper, to taste

Juice from ½ lime

1 tablespoon tomato paste

½ cup water

Taco Toppings

Chopped cilantro

Petite diced bell pepper

Thinly sliced radish

Chopped green onion

Chopped avocado

Salsa

Preheat the oven to 400 degrees. Rub coconut oil over the outside of each potato and place them onto a glass or ceramic baking dish. Bake for 30-40 minutes until they are fork tender.

Meanwhile, brown the meat in a cast iron skillet over medium heat. Add the green chilis, chili powder, oregano, garlic powder, sea salt, black pepper and lime juice and give it a good stir. Next add the tomato paste and water and stir until all ingredients are well combined.

Cut each sweet potato down the center and open to create plenty of space for toppings. Begin with the meat and continue to pile on more as much of other of the toppings listed as you like until it is a true taco masterpiece.

To keep the fun going even as you do the dishes, I encourage you to find a little Latin music and take a few spins around the kitchen. It's the perfect way to celebrate your taco night done right!

Deliciously Holistic: Inspired Favorites

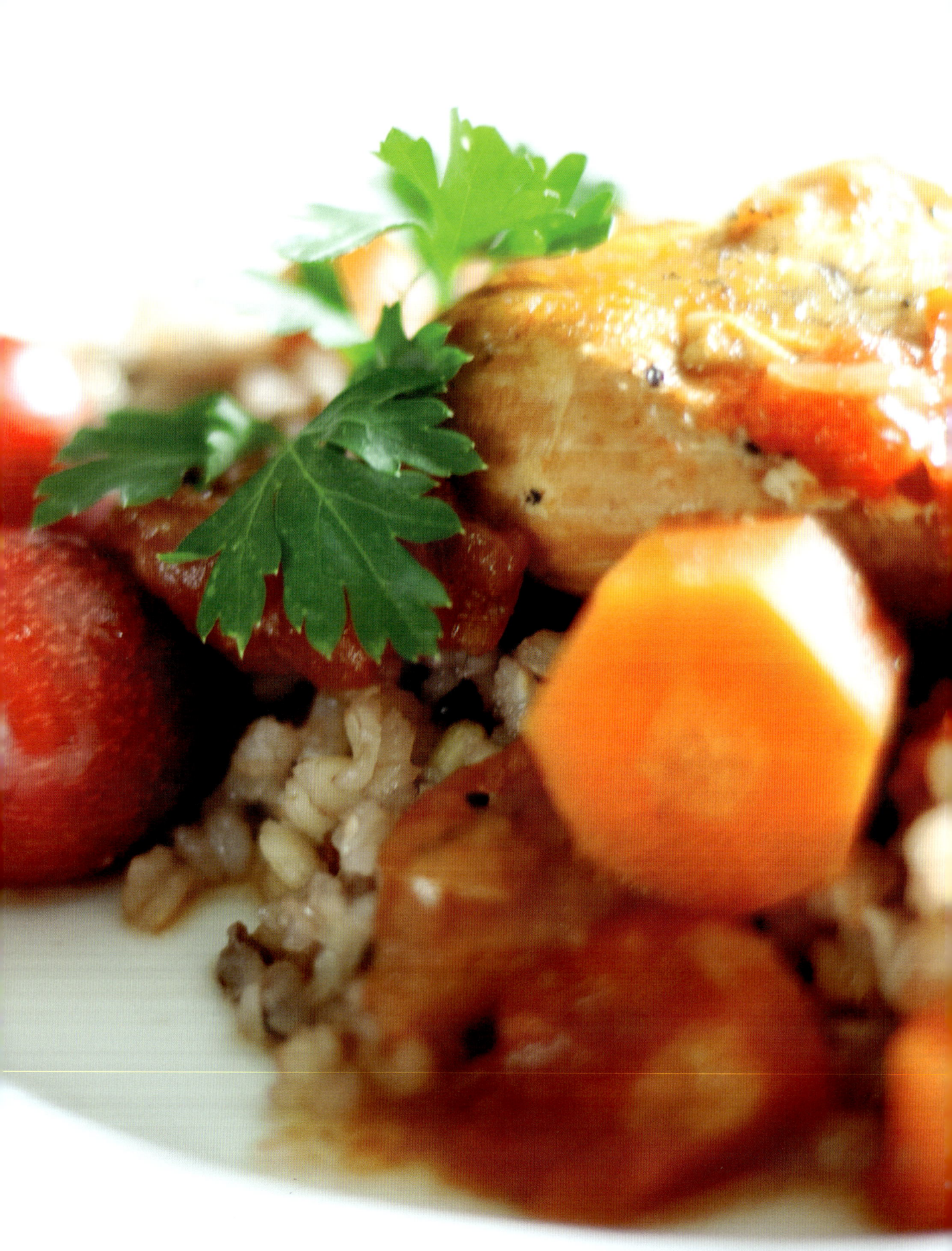

Slow-Cooked Sweetly Spiced Chicken

Throughout the years, I have heard every reason imaginable why a person is unable or unwilling to eat healthy. My favorite excuse is: "Eating healthy is just too bland. I like flavorful food way too much to make the switch." Clearly, they have never tasted MY food! This recipe is so loaded with flavor you will forget you are eating well (not that you should forget). For all of those flavor seekers out there—this one is for you! If you don't already have allspice sitting in your spice rack—go buy it! You will be making this recipe over and over again.

- 2 teaspoons coconut oil, divided
- 1 pound organic chicken breast
- Sea salt and black pepper, to taste
- 2 shallots, thinly sliced
- 2 garlic cloves, finely chopped
- 2 medium carrots, sliced into bite-sized pieces
- ½ teaspoon cinnamon
- ¼ teaspoon allspice
- 1 tablespoon freshly grated ginger root
- 1 (15-ounce) can organic diced tomatoes
- 1 cup fresh pitted cherries, halved
- 1 cup chicken or bone broth
- ½ cup fresh parsley or cilantro

Heat 1 teaspoon of coconut oil in a skillet over medium heat. Season chicken breasts on both sides with sea salt and black pepper and add to the hot pan. Cook each side for 3–5 minutes until browned but not cooked through, then place chicken in your slow cooker.

Add the second teaspoon of coconut oil and shallots to the skillet and sauté for 3 minutes. Add the garlic and cook for 1 minute more. Add shallots and garlic to the slow-cooker along with carrots, cinnamon, allspice, ginger, tomatoes, cherries, broth and a bit more sea salt and black pepper. Give everything a stir to combine, keeping the chicken at the bottom of the slow cooker. Cook on high for 3–4 hours or on low for 6–7 hours.

Once on your plate, top with cilantro or parsley and enjoy! Pairs perfectly with a sprouted wild rice blend and a mixed greens salad. Wildly flavorful, healthy dinner accomplished.

Tip: Although you could technically use powdered ginger (switch the measurement to 1 teaspoon), buying fresh ginger root is simple, affordable and beautifully fragrant. You will find it in the produce section at your grocery store, sold by the pound. Simply break off a small piece or buy a large piece and store it in the freezer for up to 2 months. Use the back of a spoon to easily scrape away the skin.

Deliciously Holistic: Inspired Favorites

Sensational Sauces & Spreads

spread the love

Pesto Please! DONE 2 WAYS

I am sucker for all things Italian—food, wine, vacations (well, I have not yet traveled there but live vicariously through friends that do). Pesto is one of those Italian staples that everyone loves and yet very few people make for themselves. I was inspired to make two versions of this deliciously versatile condiment to please all readers: one that honors the original Italian roots and another that well, cranks it up a nutritional notch. Whichever version you choose to bless those around you with, it won't disappoint. But be prepared to make a double batch; you will be spreading this stuff on everything. Buon Appetito!

Besto Pesto

- 1 cup fresh basil, tightly packed
- 1 cup fresh spinach, tightly packed
- 1 garlic clove
- 1 tablespoon freshly squeezed lemon juice
- ¼ cup pine nuts
- ¼ cup nutritional yeast
- ¼ cup olive oil
- ½ teaspoon sea salt
- ½ teaspoon black pepper

Powerhouse Pesto

- 1 cup dandelion greens, tightly packed
- ½ cup kale, ribs removed and tightly packed
- ½ cup fresh parsley, tightly packed
- 1 cup fresh basil, tightly packed
- 1 garlic clove
- ⅓ cup walnuts
- ¼ cup nutritional yeast
- 2 tablespoons freshly squeezed lemon juice
- ⅓ cup olive oil
- ½ teaspoon sea salt
- ½ teaspoon black pepper

Using a food processor, blend all ingredients until you achieve a desired consistency. Scrape down the sides with a spatula as necessary to incorporate every bit of goodness. Makes for an enticing accompaniment to carrot and celery sticks or your favorite seeded cracker.

Add a touch more olive oil to use it as a salad dressing. If you would like to turn this into a sauce for simmering or coating chicken or fish, simply stir in some broth or non-dairy milk to make it smooth and creamy.

Harness your inner Italian and get creative in your kitchen! Having Andrea Bocelli playing in the background is optional, but highly recommended.

Deliciously Holistic: Inspired Favorites

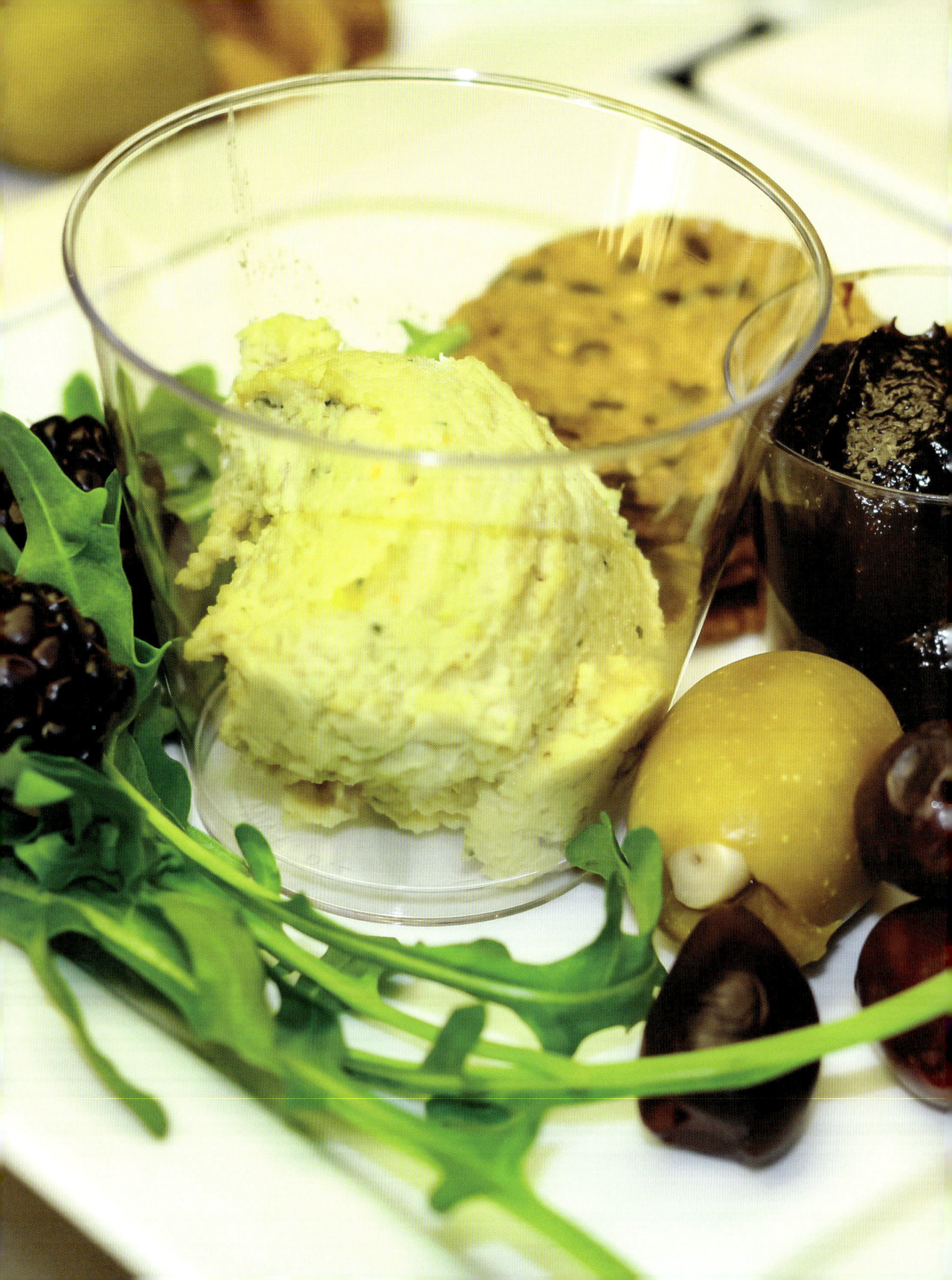

Spreadable Cashew Cheese DONE 2 WAYS

I love cheese. I have always loved cheese. There was a lot of cheese in my diet growing up, although none of it was in good form. Instead, it was processed, loaded with hormones and other chemicals, and often powdered. Yuck! Now that I have spent time learning all about what dairy does to our bodies as a whole, I felt compelled to find a way to enjoy the experience of cheese without suffering the consequences. Creamy, protein filled and lovely. Yes, please.

Lemon Thyme Cashew Cheese

- 1 cup raw cashews, soaked and rinsed
- 1 tablespoon nutritional yeast
- ⅛ teaspoon garlic powder
- 2 tablespoons fresh squeezed lemon juice
- 2 tablespoons water
- ⅛ teaspoon ground mustard
- Leaves from 6 fresh thyme stems
- Zest from 1 lemon
- Sea salt and black pepper, to taste

Smoky Cashew Cheese

- 1 cup raw cashews, soaked and rinsed
- 1 tablespoon tahini
- ⅛ teaspoon smoked paprika
- ⅛ teaspoon ground mustard
- ⅛ teaspoon onion powder
- 2 tablespoons nutritional yeast
- 4 tablespoons water

Add all ingredients to a food processor and blend until creamy. Flavors will develop the longer they have a chance to sit in the fridge.

Serve chilled or at room temperature as part of a charcuterie platter or simply with some carrot and celery sticks.

Tip: When attempting to make any style of "nut cheese," it is imperative that you soak your raw nuts for at least 1 hour. You can certainly soak them overnight if you remember to do so before your evening tea.

Deliciously Holistic: Inspired Favorites

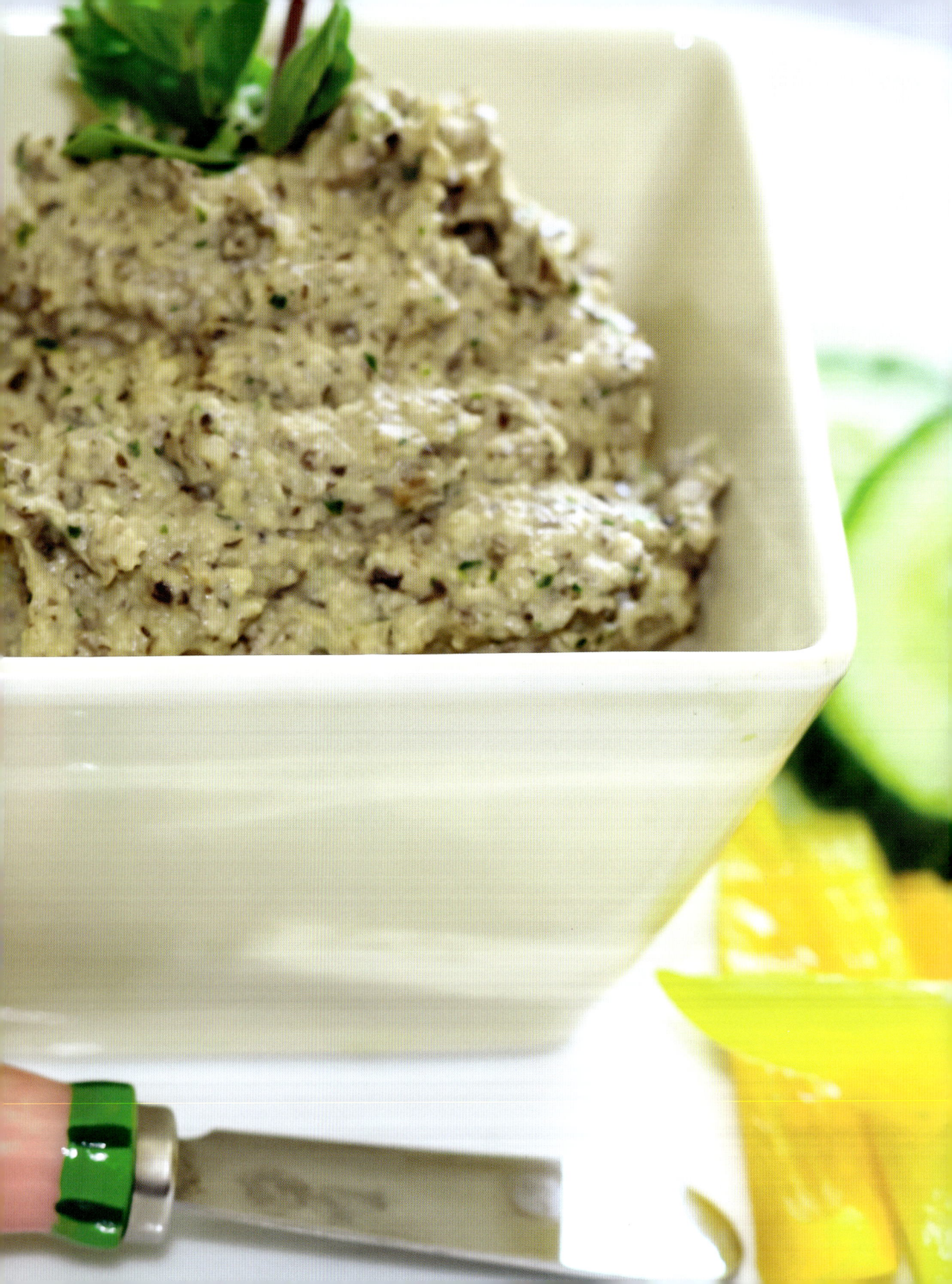

Roasted Eggplant & Wild Mushroom Dip

There is something about the process of roasting that brings out the very best in some foods. Mushrooms are certainly one of those! Go for wild mushrooms such as shitake, maitake and oyster as they provide greater health benefits than white button. Wild mushrooms also add a rich, robust flavor that will keep you going back for more. Even if you are not currently fond of mushrooms—or eggplant for that matter, give this recipe a shot. You just may find yourself to be a blossoming fan of fungus (Yep—that's what I said).

1 medium to large eggplant

16 oz. wild mushrooms *(oyster, shitake, crimini)*—**roughly chopped**

Avocado oil *(enough to lightly coat the mushrooms)*

Sea salt and black pepper, to taste

½ cup walnuts

2 garlic cloves

½ cup fresh parsley

¼ cup fresh oregano

2 tablespoons freshly squeezed lemon juice

¼ cup olive oil

¼ cup tahini

Preheat oven to 400 degrees. Place eggplant in a baking dish lined with parchment paper. Roast for 30–40 minutes until the skin gets puffy. Toss the mushrooms in enough avocado oil to give them a light coating along with some sea salt and black pepper. Add these to the oven about half way through roasting the eggplant as they will only take 15 minutes or so to roast. Toss the mushrooms once during the cooking process to ensure they don't burn.

Remove the eggplant and mushrooms from the oven and allow to cool. Once cool enough to handle, remove the skin from the eggplant and discard.

In a food processor, add mushrooms, eggplant, walnuts, garlic cloves, parsley, oregano, lemon juice, olive oil, tahini, sea salt and black pepper. Blend until ingredients are nicely incorporated. If you over blend, you will end up with a true puree. This works just fine for a dip unless you are looking for it to have a little more texture.

This will remain fresh in the fridge for up to 10 days although I have never seen it last that long when carrots sticks or gluten-free crackers are on hand.

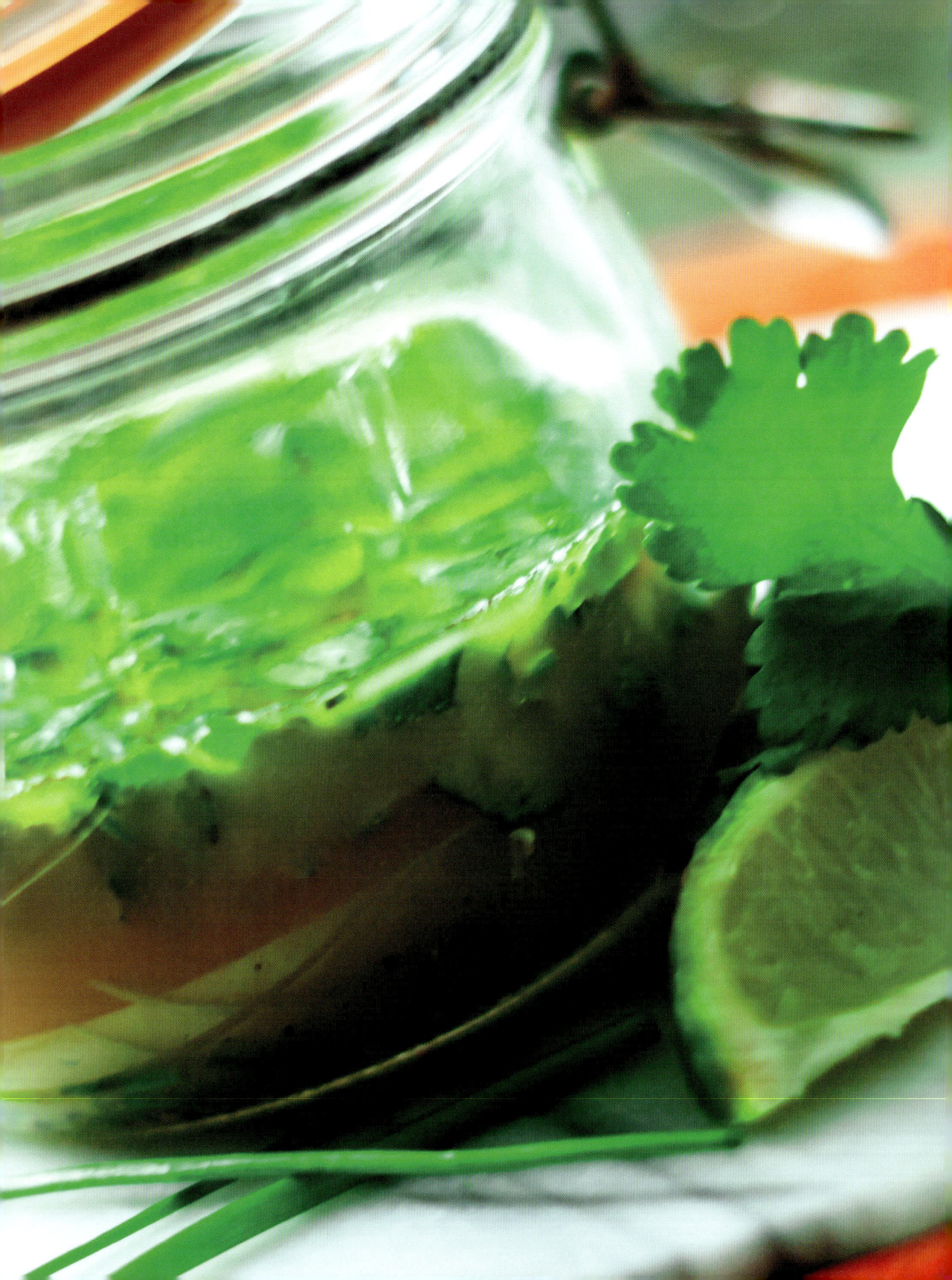

Addressing the Dressing

I often get asked if I make my own almond milk, fermented veggies, and certainly my own bone broth. The honest answer is—no, I actually don't. Could I? Should I? Of course! But even I have to pick and choose how I spend my own 24 hours each day. If I am making every single meal, snack and morning smoothie for four people from scratch seven days a week, there would be no time left to exercise, meditate or perhaps offer my husband a moment of my day. Where is the balance in that? There is one item however that I simply will not purchase pre-made as I find it to be nutritionally ridiculous—and that product is salad dressing. Although there are a few exceptions currently popping up at the grocery store, most salad dressings still consist of refined sugars, sub-par oils and other processed junk; not to mention it is criminally expensive for what is in the bottle. If you are following the recipes in this book, you will never need to buy dressing again as you already have everything you need waiting there in your kitchen.

Summertime Cilantro Lime Dressing

This recipe is fresh, bright and leaves you wanting more. Sounds like summer, does it not?

- ¾ cup olive oil
- Juice from 1 lime
- ½ cup fresh cilantro, chopped
- 2 tablespoons chives, finely chopped
- Sea salt and black pepper, to taste

Delicious Dry-Herb Dressing

You may think you are cutting a nutritional corner by using dried herbs instead of fresh, but this is certainly not the case. In fact, some herbs provide a bigger nutritional punch when they have been dried.

- ¾ cup extra virgin olive oil
- ¼ cup red wine vinegar
- 1 teaspoon dried basil
- 1 teaspoon dried thyme
- 1 teaspoon dried oregano
- 1 teaspoon garlic powder
- ¼ teaspoon crushed red pepper
- Sea salt and black pepper, to taste
- A squeeze of fresh lemon juice (optional—if you happen to have one on hand)

Add all ingredients to a mason jar or any other glass jar with a tight-fitting lid. Shake well and conservatively pour over your favorite salad. (You can always add more dressing, tougher to take away when you have added too much.) Store leftovers in the refrigerator.

Wellness is not about perfection; it is about progress. Even if the only thing you make from scratch today is your salad dressing, consider it a great success—and tomorrow you will have another.

Deliciously Holistic: Inspired Favorites

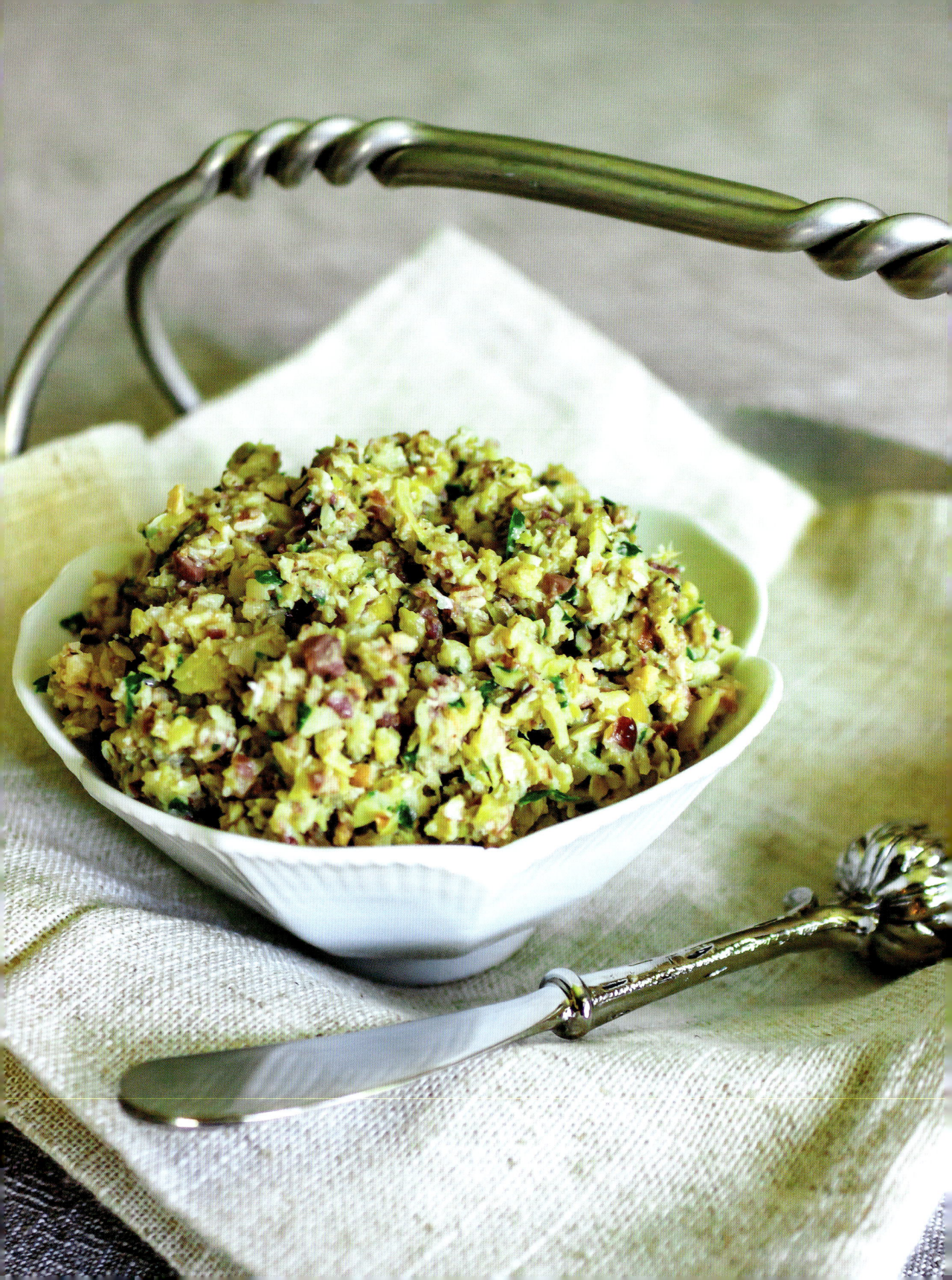

Olive a Good Tapenade

A tapenade is a fancy French term for a spread traditionally made of olives, capers and olive oil. Since I'm continuously inspired by the way the rest of the world eats, I decided to celebrate the French side of my heritage while staying true to my desire for superior nutrition. While there is certainly nothing wrong with simply blending olives, capers and olive oil to develop a multi-functional condiment, why not toss in a few more ingredients and give those fancy French folks a run for their franc. (Actually, they have switched to the euro—but you knew that.)

8 ounces artichoke hearts (*I prefer previously frozen but you can use jarred as long as they are drained and patted dry*)

20 Greek olives, pitted (*any blend of colors you like*)

1 tablespoon capers

1 garlic clove, chopped

¼ cup pecans

1 tablespoon fresh parsley

1 teaspoon fresh thyme

Juice from ½ lemon

1 tablespoon olive oil

Sea salt and black pepper, to taste

Add all ingredients to a food processor and pulse until you receive the desired consistency. Scrape down the sides as necessary.

Store in the refrigerator for up to one week.

Spread on anything in need of a little French flair.

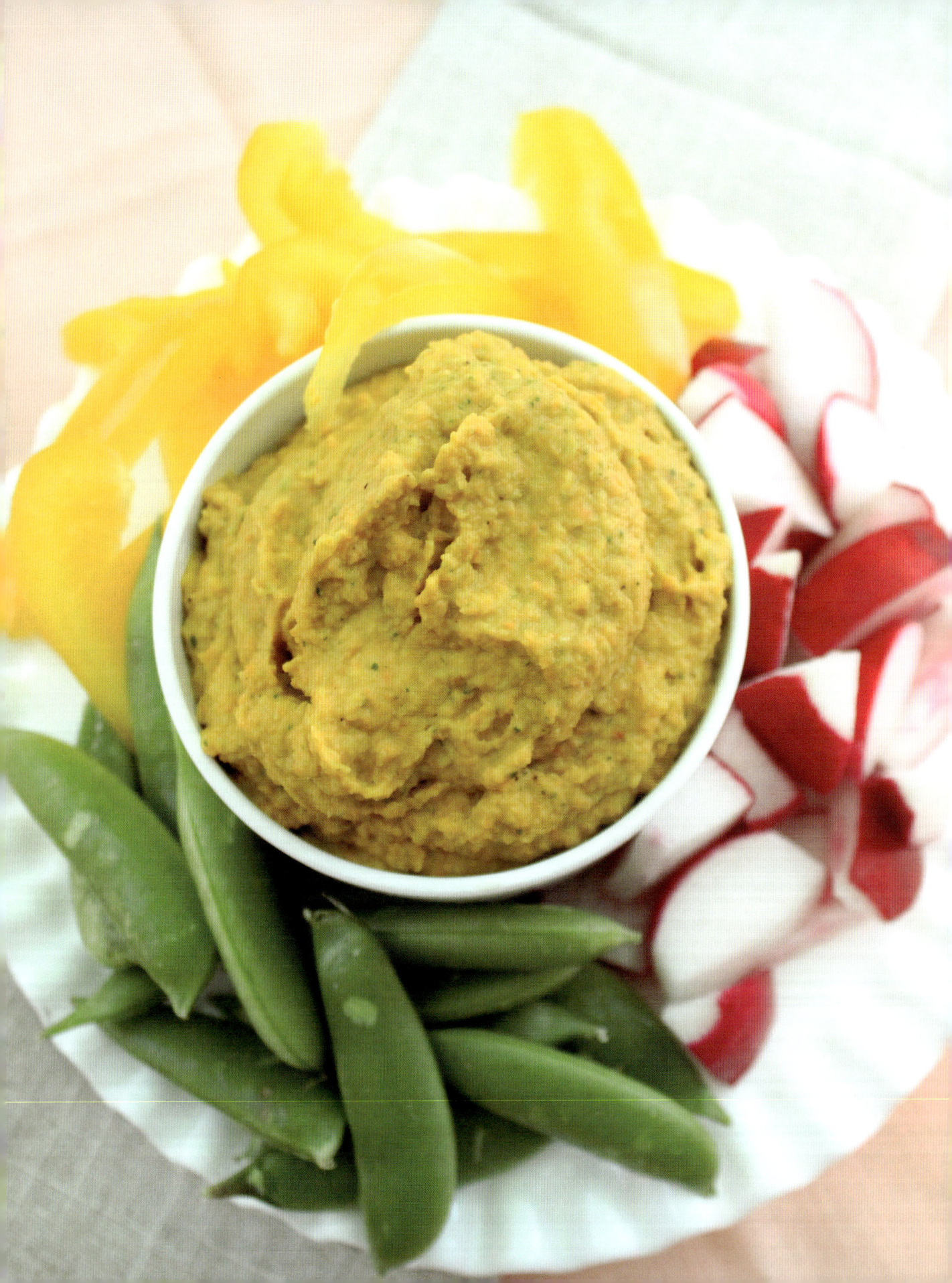

Snack on this!
Roasted Carrot & White Bean Hummus

The most common void in a new client's diet is vegetables. When I inquire about snacking habits, the answer typically includes chips, popcorn, muffins, cookies and yes, even candy. A desire for a snack is not something that needs to be ignored or denied; rather it is the definition of a snack that needs tweaking. If your body is truly hungry (assuming you are not snacking out of boredom), you are most likely depleted of necessary nutrients and calories that your body requires to keep up with your busy day. I have discovered that overall, people are willing to eat vegetables as a snack if there is something flavorful to dip it in. Try this recipe with your favorite fresh vegetables and give your body the type of snack it is actually craving.

2 large carrots, peeled and chopped into 1–1 ½ inch chunks

1 yellow onion, sliced

2 garlic cloves

2 tablespoons avocado oil, divided

Sea salt and black pepper, to taste

½ cup fresh parsley leaves

1 (15-ounce) can organic cannellini or white northern beans, drained and rinsed

1 tablespoon tahini

Juice from ½ lemon

Preheat oven to 400 degrees.

Place carrots, onion and garlic on a baking sheet and drizzle with one tablespoon of avocado oil. Sprinkle on some sea salt and black pepper and toss to coat. Place in the oven to roast for 18–20 minutes or until the carrots are soft.

Add the veggies to a food processor along with the parsley, beans, tahini, lemon juice, and one tablespoon of avocado oil. Blend until smooth. Give it a taste test to see if it requires a bit more sea salt or black pepper and blend again if necessary.

If you are the type to crave spicy foods, be sure to add a few dashes of hot sauce or some crushed red pepper before serving. Best served chilled.

I certainly don't spend my days snacking on plain carrots and celery sticks and I don't expect any of my clients to either. I do expect they will consume their veggies on a regular basis with mindful dips and spreads to fully enjoy the experience of eating well.

Deliciously Holistic: Inspired Favorites

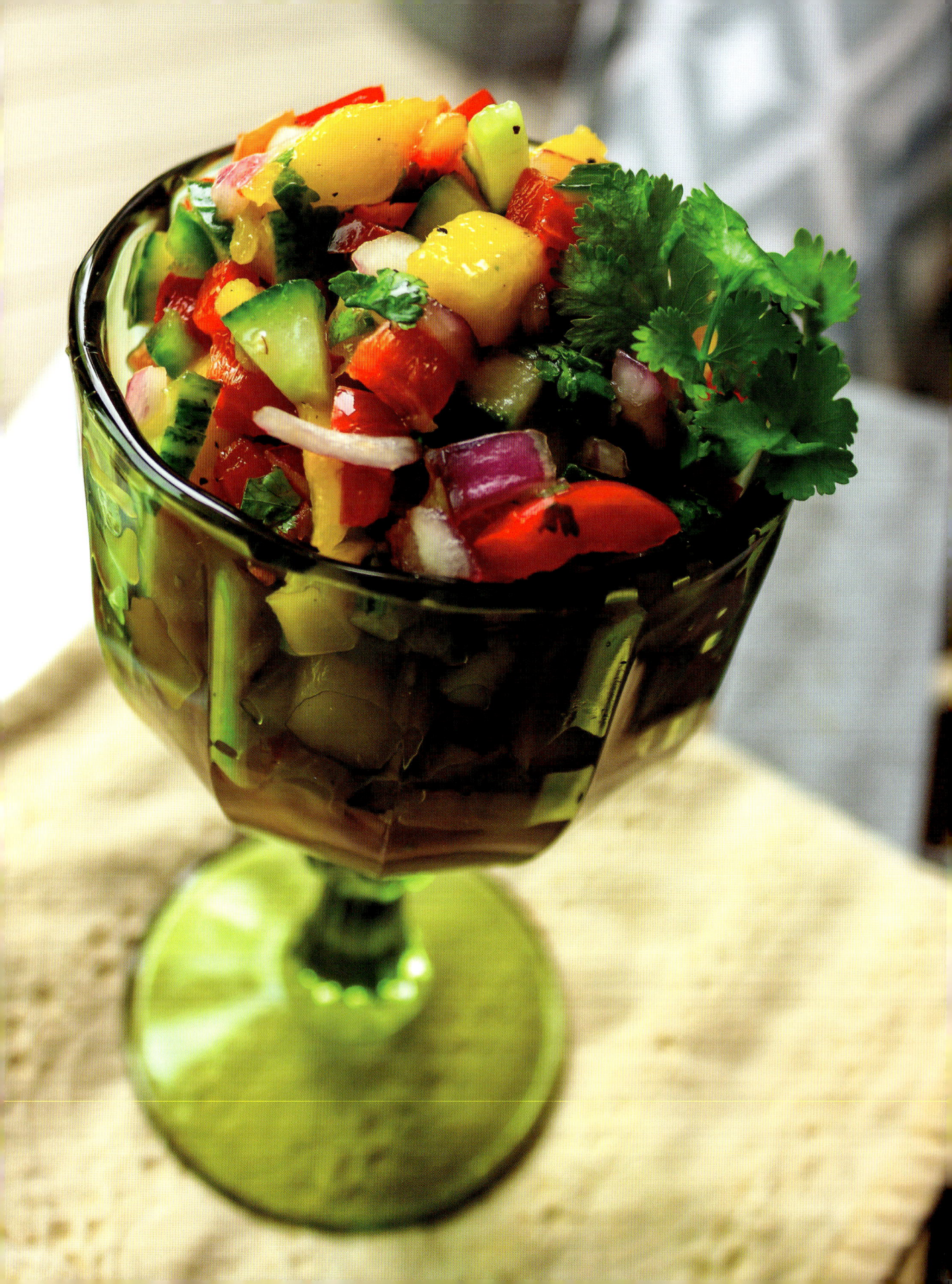

Ella's Favorite Mango Salsa

Everyone has their favorite salsa. Some like the heat and some like it sweet. Some prefer it chunky while others go for the thin, saucy variety. In my house, everyone likes something a little different. And in my quest to find a store-bought family favorite, I have discovered one common ingredient among them all: SUGAR. Even the extra hot varieties almost always have some type of added sweetener which I can only assume is to balance the flavor and act as a preservative. Since my daughter Ella can blow through salsa by the bucket full, it was necessary that I create a recipe that satisfies her sweet tooth without compromising her health. This recipe allows you to be like Ella and enjoy it like no one is watching.

1 mango, diced *(should yield 1–1 ½ cups)*

1 small bell pepper, seeded and petite diced

¾ cup English *(seedless)* **cucumber, petite diced**

½ cup red onion, petite diced

1 tablespoon jalapeño, seeded and petite diced

1 cup fresh cilantro leaves, chopped

Juice from ½ lime

Sea salt and black pepper, to taste

Add all ingredients to a large bowl and stir to combine. Although the flavor is instantly fantastic, if you allow it to sit in the refrigerator for at least 20 minutes it will be even better.

This recipe will give you a very chunky salsa. If you prefer your salsa more like a puree, simply add it to a blender and pulse until you reach your desired consistency.

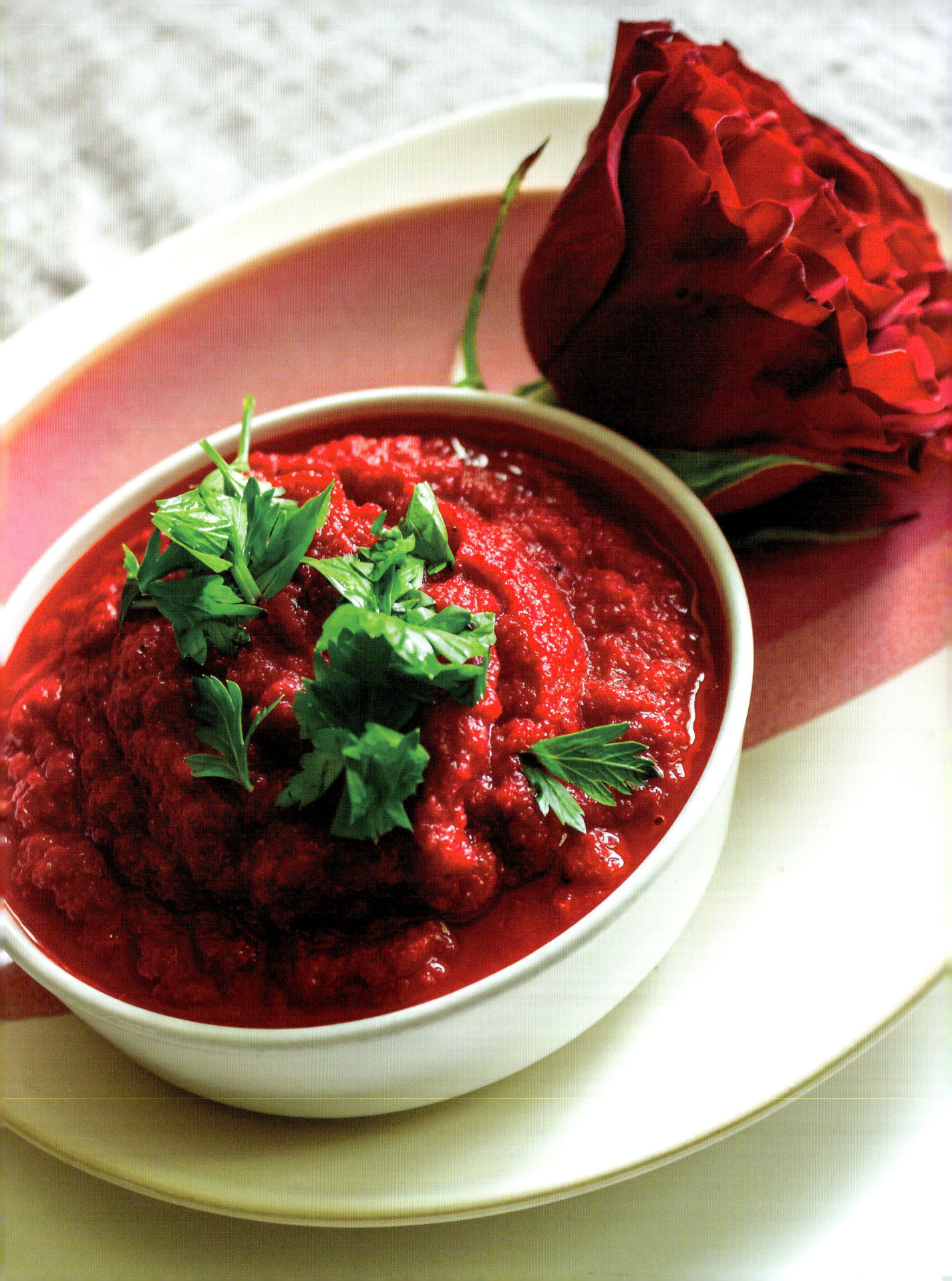

Valentine Marinara

Red has always been associated with hearts and love. To give your heart what it really loves, eat plenty of red foods. Tomatoes and beets are just two of the red foods that help to promote a healthy functioning heart. This February, rather than giving your valentine a box of harmful sugary treats, opt for spending a little extra time in the kitchen and make something extra special. This recipe is admittedly more labor intensive than my usual creations, but your heart will be so appreciative of your efforts.

4 medium beets *(each should be about 2 inches)*

2–3 tablespoons avocado oil, divided

Sea salt and black pepper, to taste

1 small cauliflower, chopped into approximately 1–inch pieces

1 small yellow onion, sliced

4 garlic cloves

1 teaspoon dried oregano

1 teaspoon dried basil

1 (28-ounce) can crushed tomatoes

⅓ cup Cabernet *(or other dark red wine)*

⅓ cup vegetable broth

Line a glass or ceramic baking dish with parchment paper and preheat the oven to 400 degrees. If you purchase your beets with the tops still attached, simply cut the stems off leaving just enough to grab on to and keep the tails intact. Rub a thin layer of avocado oil over each beet, sprinkle with sea salt and place on the parchment paper lined pan. Roast for 45–55 minutes or until you can easily insert a knife into the center of each beet. Allow to cool slightly. Use the knife to help remove the skins and quarter each beet. These will *(temporarily)* stain your hands, so handle with care or use gloves.

While the beets are roasting, add the cauliflower, onion and garlic to a second baking dish and sprinkle on oregano, basil, sea salt and black pepper. Add the remaining avocado oil and toss well to coat. Place in the oven alongside the beets and roast for 20–25 minutes or until the cauliflower is soft and golden.

In a large saucepan, add the tomatoes, beets and other roasted veggies along with the wine and broth and blend with an immersion blender until you achieve your desired marinara consistency. Your sauce will now have a gorgeous pink hue! Bring to a simmer and allow to cook for 20–30 minutes stirring occasionally. Give it a little taste test and add more oregano, basil, sea salt or black pepper if necessary. Serve as an appetizer with a nut flour bread for dipping or as an entrée on top of some spiralized zucchini.

A glass of dark red wine is also considered a heart healthy choice and just happens to pair nicely with a romantic dinner at home.

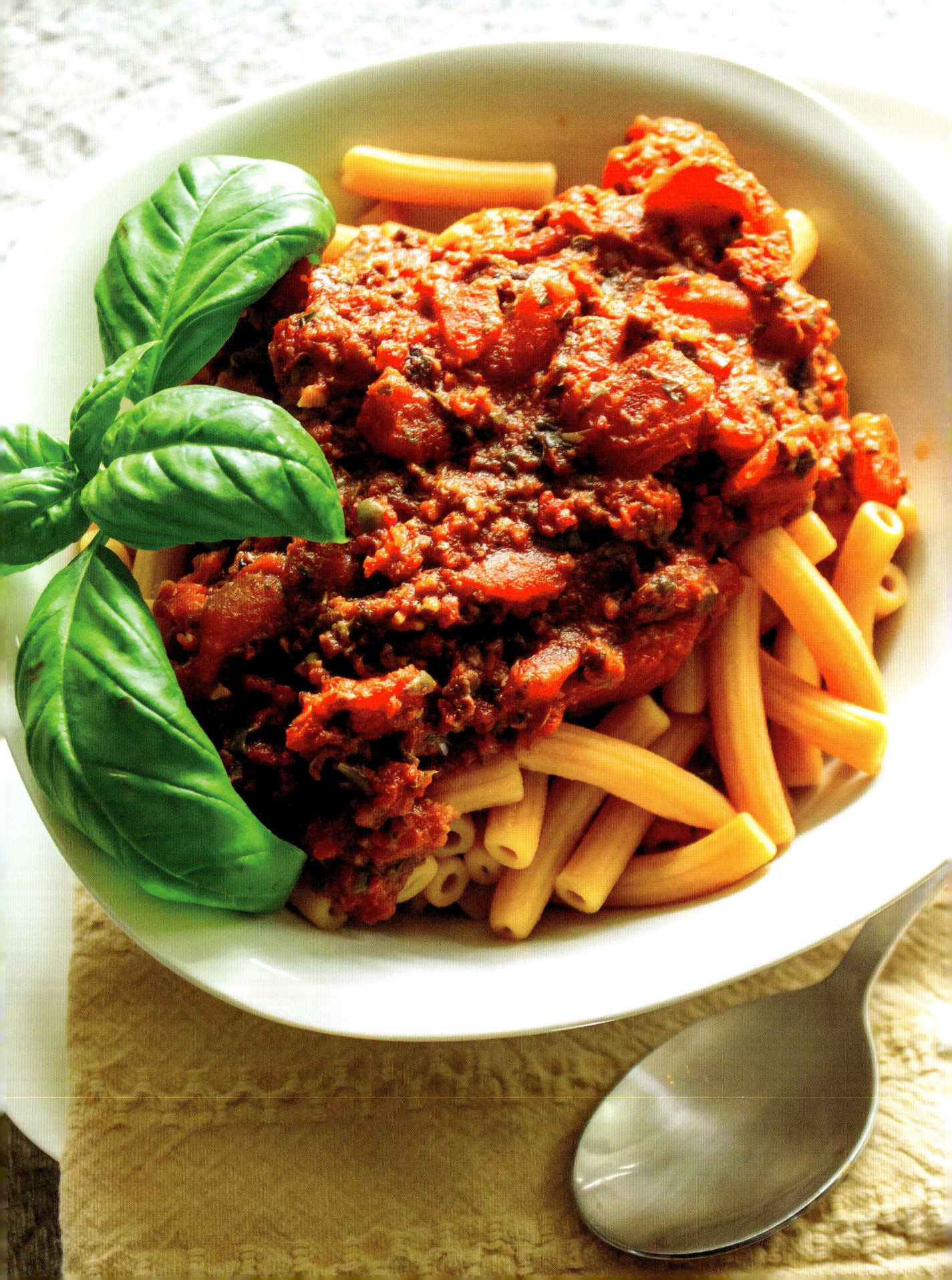

Accent Inspiring Puttanesca

Although my husband, Brian, is not fan of raw tomato, when cooked and blended into a sweet sauce he suddenly becomes 100 percent Italian. While he is of some Italian descent, somehow when enough garlic and fresh basil is involved, a full accent comes rolling off his tongue. For those of you who are real Italians, you may notice that I have left out a common ingredient in this recipe—the anchovies. Although anchovies are incredibly good for you and are fairly easy to find, I didn't want any new holistic home chef to be put off by having to include a few flat fish. If you are a true Italian or are ready to play one in your kitchen, by all means—add them in!

1 cup fresh basil, well packed

1 cup fresh parsley

2 garlic cloves

½ cup Kalamata olives, pitted and drained

1 ½ tablespoons capers, drained

½ cup sun-dried tomatoes

Sea salt and black pepper, to taste

1 *(28-ounce)* **can organic crushed tomatoes**

1 *(15-ounce)* **can organic diced tomatoes**

¼ teaspoon crushed red pepper

Using a food processor, first place the basil and parsley in the bottom and add the garlic, olives, capers and sun-dried tomatoes on top. Season with a bit of sea salt and black pepper and blend for just a few second to combine. Scrape down the sides and blend for a few seconds more.

Pour the crushed tomatoes, diced tomatoes, crushed red pepper and more sea salt and black pepper in a medium sauce pan. Next add the olive, caper, garlic and herb mixture and stir well to combine. Cover and bring to a simmer. Allow the sauce to cook for 20–30 minutes, stirring occasionally.

Use this sauce to top spaghetti squash or lentil pasta and sprinkle on a little nutritional yeast in place of the Parmesan cheese. It is a surprisingly satisfying substitution.

Chi mangia bene, vive bene—which is Italian for, "Who eats well, lives well"!

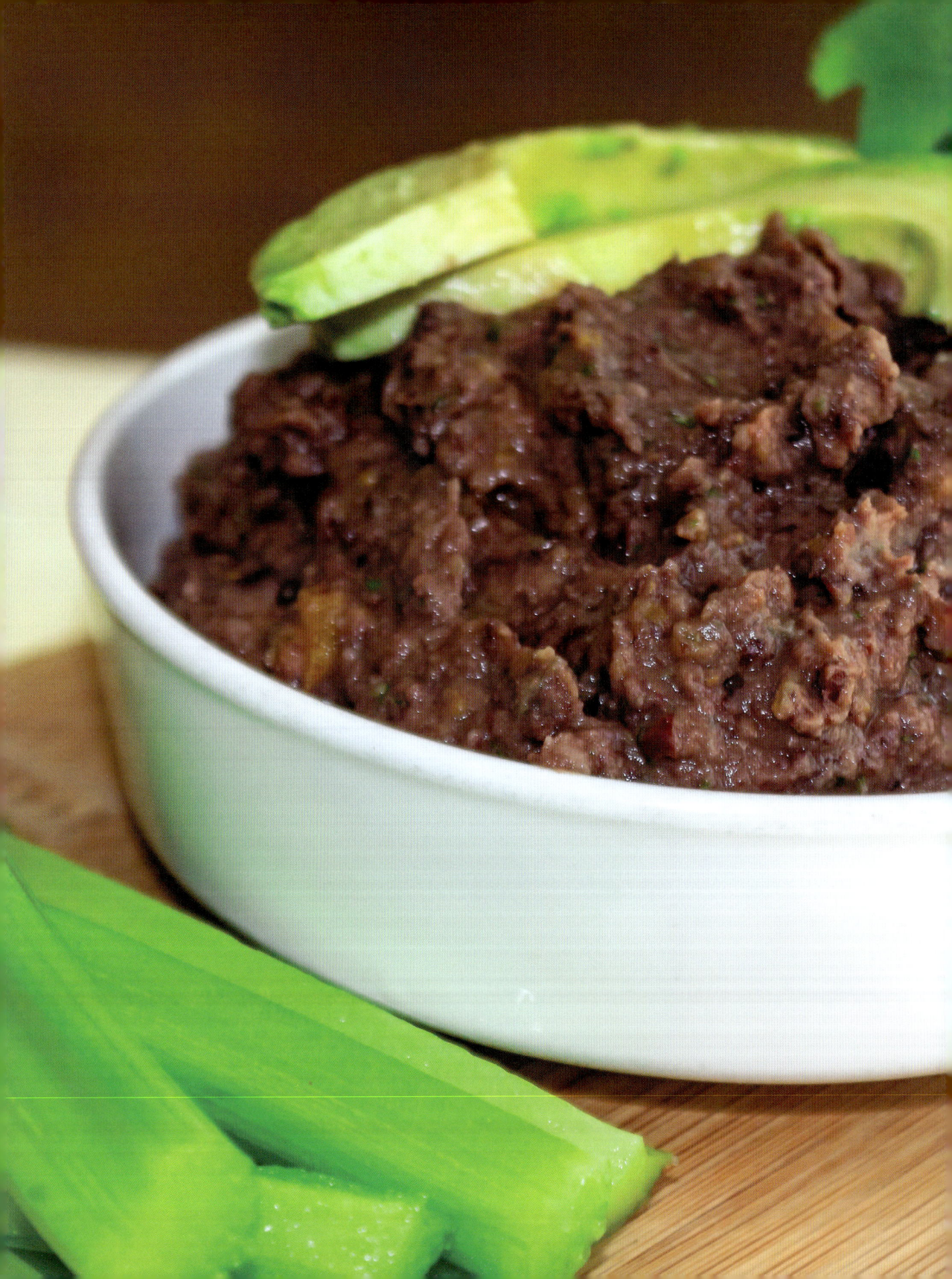

Bangin' Black Bean Dip

Our hometown is truly a destination spot. It is known for its many lakes, its spectacular summer fireworks display, and certainly its focus on family fun. But perhaps the most famous of destinations in Lake Orion is the ever-popular Mexican restaurant right in the heart of downtown. Over the years I have often wondered why this place is always packed with happy patrons. Is it the service? The ambiance? The margaritas? Being the food-focused gal that I am, I have come to determine that it is the traditional Mexican flavors that everyone adores. This recipe offers all of the fun and flavor you desire without having to wait for a table.

2 (15-ounce) cans organic black beans, drained and rinsed

¼ cup organic canned green chilis

½ cup jarred fire-roasted bell pepper

1 tablespoon jalapeño, diced

1 teaspoon cumin

½ freshly squeezed lime

½ cup fresh cilantro

Sea salt and black pepper, to taste

Add all ingredients to a food processor and pulse until you achieve the desired consistency. Top with a few slices of avocado and serve with plenty of veggie sticks for dipping.

If you ever find yourself visiting our hometown hot spot, be sure to ask Dave the bartender to make your margarita "Valerie style." He will leave out the sugar-filled sour mix and substitute it with a splash of club soda and plenty of freshly squeezed citrus.

Perfect Party Favorites

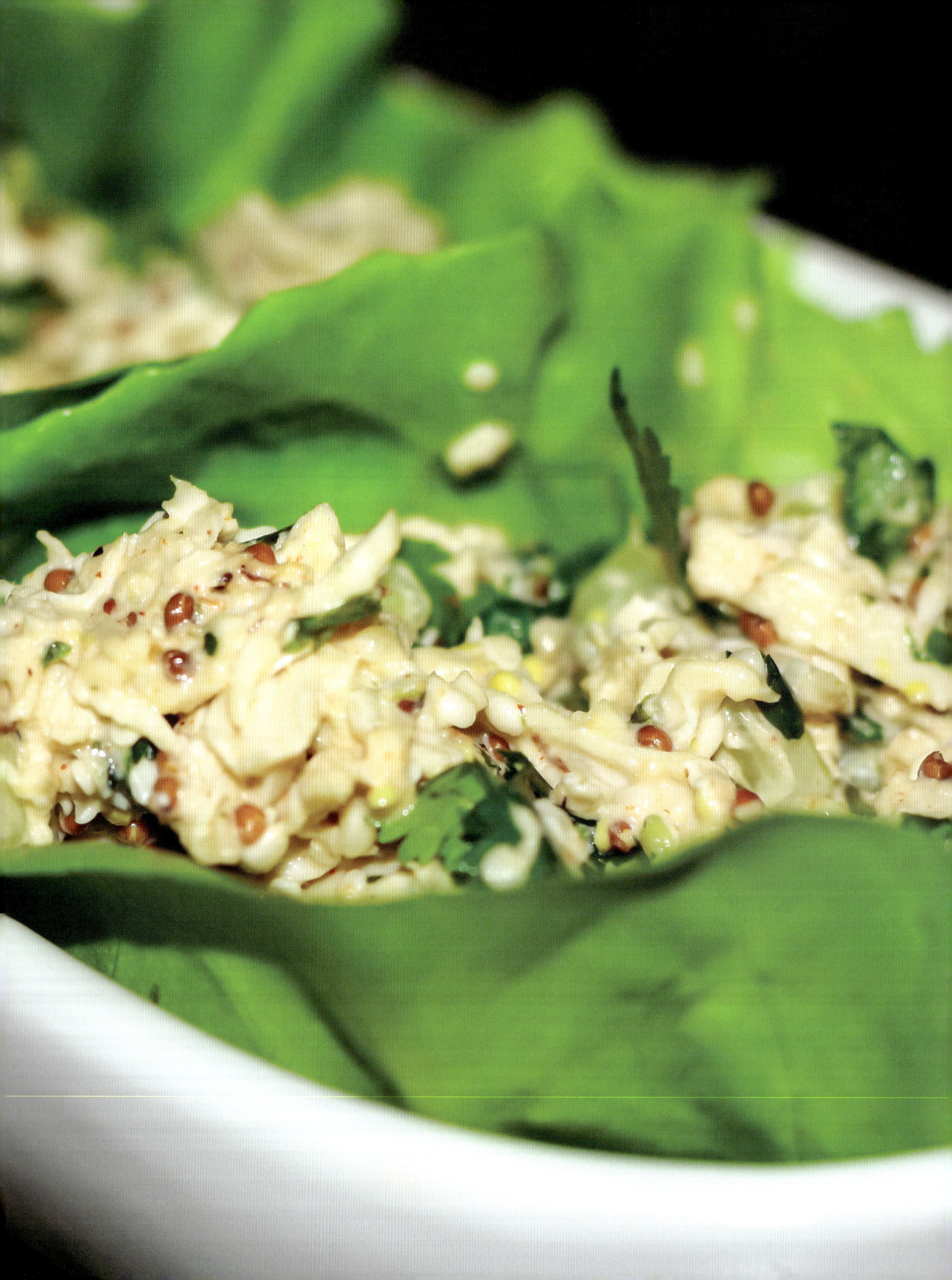

Kicked up Chicken Salad in Lettuce Cups

Never in my wildest dreams (proudly, yes—I do dream of food often) did I ever imagine I would be including a recipe for chicken salad in any of my cookbooks. Before making it myself, I had only ever experienced this dish as a massive sea of mayo with a little chicken and bits of celery served on white bread or perhaps a croissant. Hardly a nutritionist's go-to meal. When these types of recipes cross my path a few too many times, it inspires me to create something worthy of the Deliciously Holistic name.

1 ½ cups chicken or vegetable broth

1 pound organic chicken breast

½ cup fresh cilantro, chopped and tightly packed

1 cup celery, diced

¼ cup green onion, chopped

¼ cup avocado oil mayo *(avoid traditional mayo made with canola oil as it is typically genetically modified and is not well received by the body)*

⅛ cup whole grain mustard

¼ cup hemp seed

1 ½ teaspoons Cajun or blackened seasoning

1 tablespoon freshly squeezed lemon juice

Endive, Bibb lettuce or romaine leaves for serving

Sea salt and black pepper, to taste

In a medium-sized pot, add the broth and chicken breast, and cook covered over medium heat until the chicken is thoroughly cooked and no longer pink. Remove from the pot and allow to the chicken to cool. Chop chicken into bite sized pieces or pull apart with two forks if you preferred shredded chicken for this dish.

In a large glass or ceramic bowl, combine all ingredients. For the best results, place in the refrigerator for one hour to allow all the flavors to marry. For those who really like things kicked up, add a few dashes of your favorite hot sauce next or top with sliced jalapeño.

Scoop the salad onto endive, romaine or Bibb lettuce leaves, and have fun eating each portion with your hands while dining al fresco.

Tip : Using leftover rotisserie or baked chicken breast and thigh meat works great for this recipe too!

Deliciously Holistic: Inspired Favorites

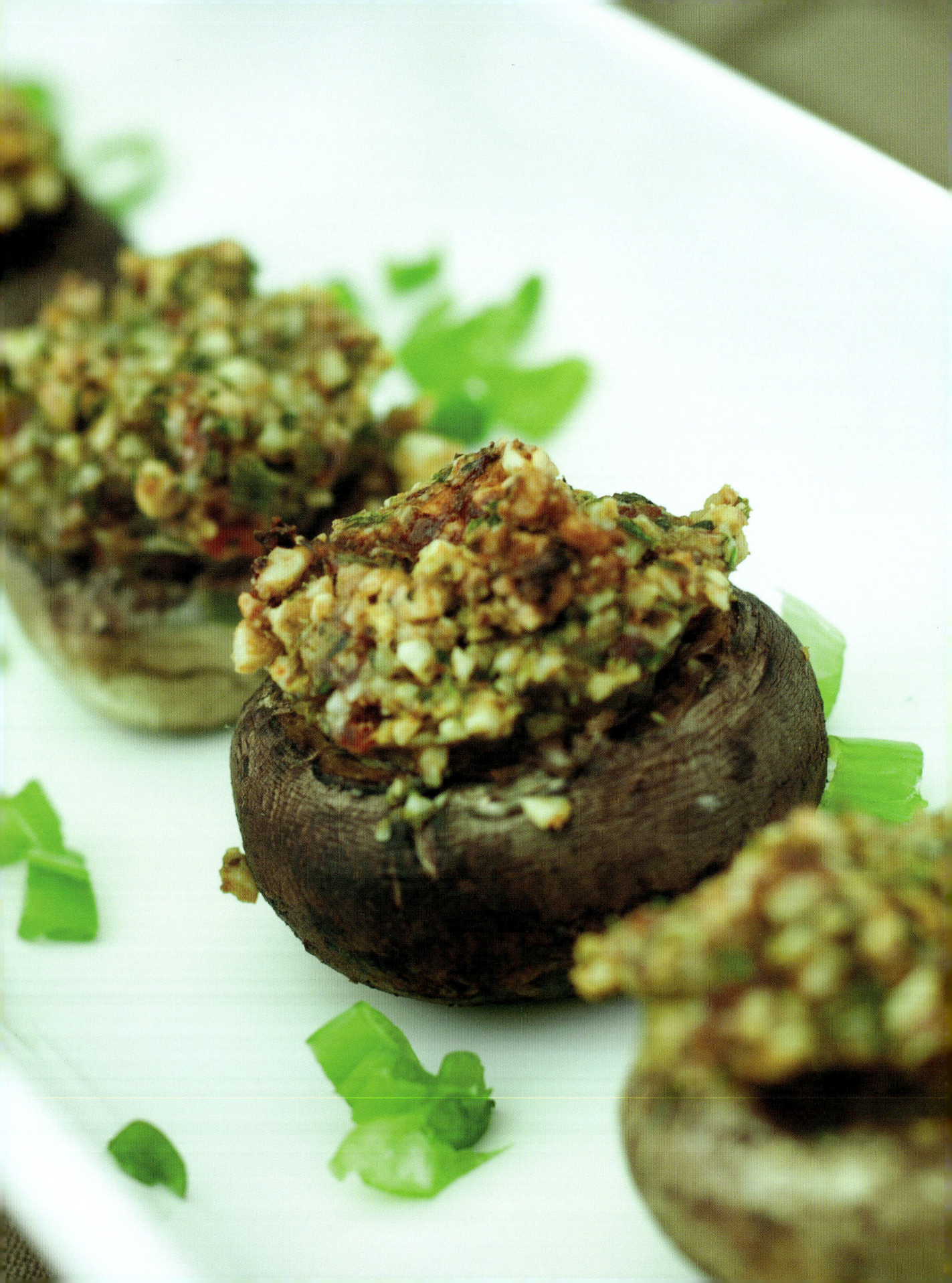

Not Quite Noah's Stuffed Mushrooms

When my son was three years old, he came up with the idea of stuffing hash browns into a mushroom cap. Quite honestly, I had never bothered to stuff a mushroom before then so I gave it a shot. Although that recipe is reserved for the next book, I decided to evolve the concept to suit my readers this time around. My version offers a simple way to pack oodles of nutritious flavor into one bite-sized little package. Whether you are using it as an appetizer for a crowd or simply want an easy-to-grab snack waiting for you in the fridge, these little guys will not disappoint. As for my own little guy who is not so little anymore, he still loves a stuffed mushroom—with or without the hash browns.

16 ounces baby Portabella or white button mushrooms

1–2 garlic cloves

½ cup chives or green onions

¼ cup sun-dried tomatoes

½ cup fresh basil

½ cup fresh parsley

¼ cup nutritional yeast

½ cup cashews

Sea salt and black pepper, to taste

Clean the mushrooms with a damp paper towel, scoop out the stems, and set in a baking dish lightly coated with coconut oil or lined with parchment paper. If you are like me, you will save your stems in the freezer with other discarded veggie ends and make vegetable broth with the collection.

Combine remaining ingredients in a food processor or very finely chop everything by hand and mix them all together in a bowl.

Stuff each mushroom with the mix and bake in a 375-degree oven about 25 minutes or until the mushrooms are soft.

These are so flavorful they can be enjoyed warm, room temperature or even cold out of the refrigerator. I have yet to discover if they freeze well; they are long gone before I ever get the opportunity to try.

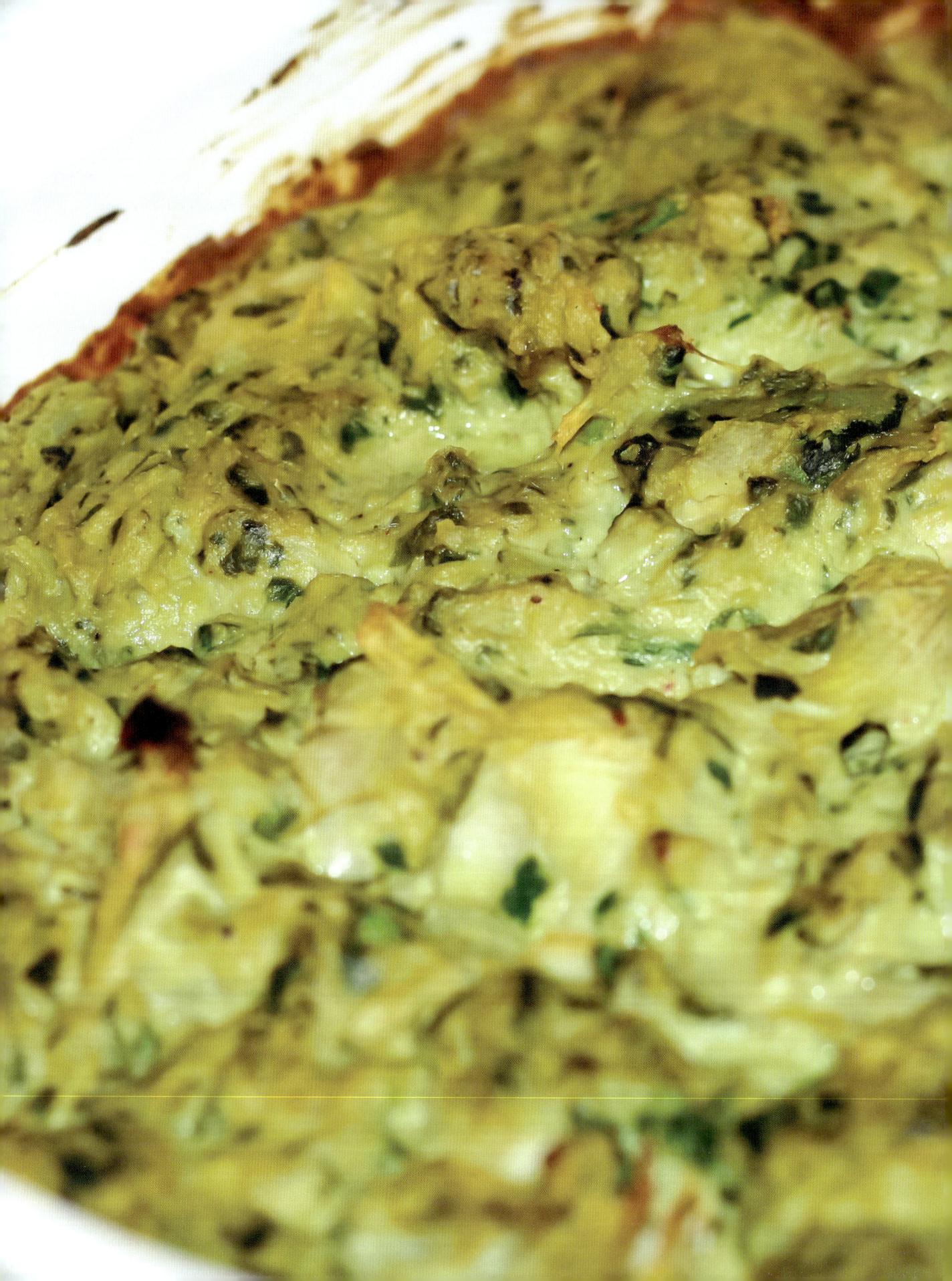

Let Them Eat Artichoke Dip

I first encountered this classic appetizer as a teenager while dining out with friends at a local chain restaurant. Although it tasted creamy and delicious, the obscene amounts of cream cheese and Parmesan always left me feeling sluggish and bloated. I decided to keep the best parts of this recipe and give the rest a necessary upgrade, making both the flavor and nutritional value worthy of this book. Go ahead and eat like you did as a teenager (just be sure to follow the instructions below, of course).

½ cup cashews

¾ cup non-dairy milk *(I like almond for this recipe)*

Juice from ½ lemon

1–2 garlic cloves *(depending on size and your taste)*

1 teaspoon sea salt

Black pepper to taste

1 teaspoon ground mustard powder

¼ cup nutritional yeast

¼ teaspoon crushed red pepper

12 oz artichoke hearts, chopped *(can use previously frozen or jarred hearts that have been drained)*

2 cups fresh spinach leaves, chopped

2 tablespoons fresh chives, chopped

Preheat oven to 425 degrees.

Using a blender, add cashews, milk, lemon juice, garlic, sea salt, black pepper, dry mustard, nutritional yeast and crushed red pepper. Blend until very smooth—not just blended. It should resemble a thick cream-based sauce or soup. Add this sauce to the baking dish along with the artichokes, spinach and chives and stir to combine. Bake for 20–25 minutes covered or uncovered if you would like the top to be golden brown.

Serve with your favorite gluten-free crackers and plenty of carrot, bell pepper and celery sticks.

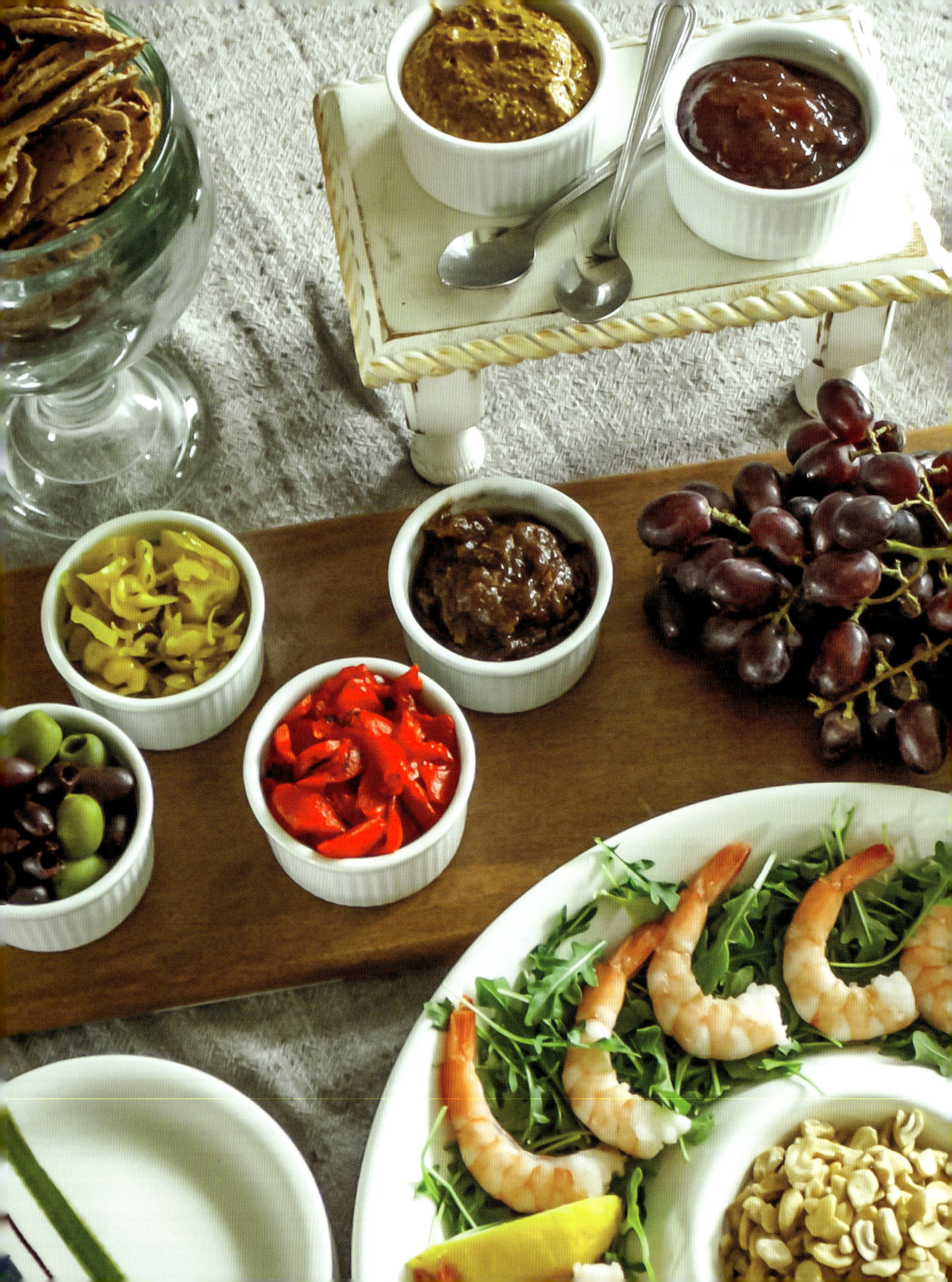

Taste of the Town

It wasn't until I was in college that I learned the art of the road trip. After many years, and many memorable trips behind me, I have discovered that most towns will have a destination street or streets where you are encouraged to shop, eat and repeat—and I am only too happy to oblige. This dinner came out of the unique and specially crafted goodies that one can only find when you talk to the locals and diligently read your labels. This meal is always a crowd favorite (even if the crowd only consists of the people who live under my own roof). It is simple but decadent and loaded with nutrition without any fuss. Pick a little of this then a little of that. Each bite is unique in flavor, texture and fun. Whether you are dining for one or have a true crowd coming to eat, this concept should be added to your culinary repertoire. And when you run out of goodies, you know it's time to hit the road again.

Using little bowls and plates, create a spread on your dinner table including any of the following:

- **Sun-dried tomatoes**
- **Marinated artichoke hearts**
- **Pickled asparagus, green beans, cauliflower or Brussels sprouts**
- **Roasted red peppers**
- **Pickles**
- **Greek olives**
- **Sweet or hot pepperoncini**
- **Pesto**
- **Salsa**
- **Onion or pepper preserves**
- **Honey, Dijon or other unique mustards**
- **Hot sauce**
- **Fresh spinach or arugula**
- **Berries, cherries or sliced peaches**
- **Wild caught shrimp or smoked salmon**
- **Cashews, walnuts, pistachios or almonds**
- **Nuts or seed crackers for building your unique creations**

Although most of the items listed above were discovered on a road trip, you can easily find many of the same unique items in the international aisle of your grocery store.

Another option is to hit a specialty or gourmet market in your own hometown to find a few delicious treasures for your fun and easy dinner spread. Always read your labels to make sure you are getting premium ingredients and not sugars, starches, and artificial colors.

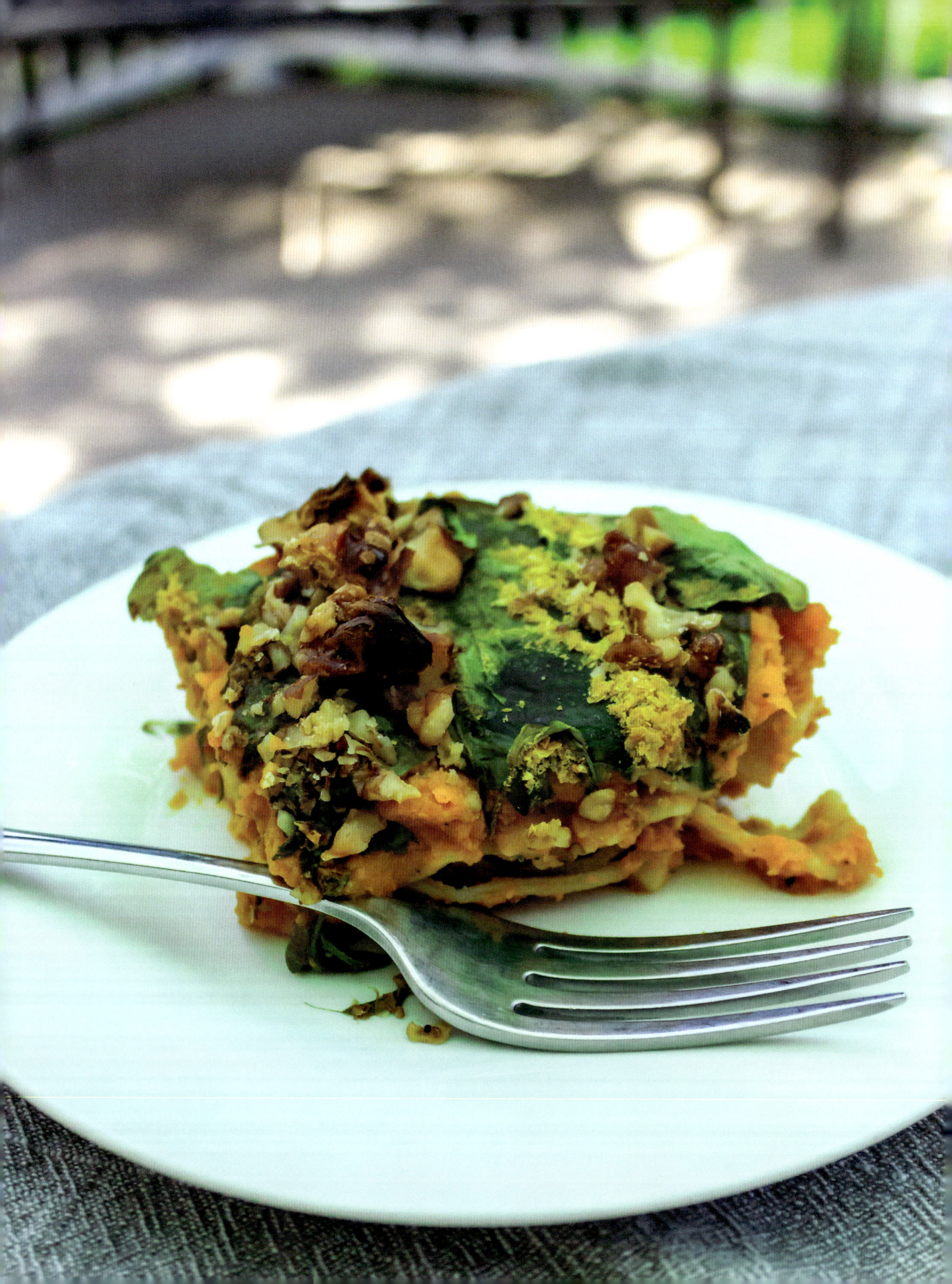

Beauteous Butternut Squash Lasagna

Some eat to live, and some live to eat...and then there are folks like me who do both. This recipe is a perfect blend of necessary nutrients and indulgent comfort that serves to satisfy every type of appetite. Now, what's more beauteous than that?

1 medium (1 ½–2 pound) butternut squash

2 tablespoons coconut oil, divided

1 large yellow onion, cut into thick slices

4 large carrots, peeled and cut into 1-inch chunks

¾ teaspoon ground sage

¾ teaspoon dried oregano

Sea salt and black pepper, to taste

1 ½ cups unsweetened non-dairy milk

1 (10-ounce) package of gluten-free lasagna noodles *(preferably brown rice or quinoa)*

10 ounces fresh spinach

1 ½ cups chopped walnuts

¼ cup nutritional yeast

Preheat oven to 400 degrees. Cut the squash lengthwise in half, scoop out the seeds and discard. Place squash skin side down on a baking sheet or glass pan. Rub 1 tablespoon of coconut oil over the inside of the squash and season with sea salt and pepper. Place into the oven to begin roasting.

Add the onion and carrot to a second glass or ceramic baking dish and sprinkle on the sage, oregano, sea salt, black pepper and 1 tablespoon of coconut oil. Toss well to coat and add to the oven to roast alongside the squash. Roast for about 20 minutes or until the carrots are fork tender. Remove from the oven and set aside. The squash may take up to 40–45 minutes total to be fully roasted. Once the squash is supremely soft, remove it from the oven and allow it to cool long enough to handle without burning yourself.

Scoop the squash away from its flesh and add to a blender along with the carrot and onion mixture and the non-dairy milk. Blend long enough to create a creamy sauce.

Using a 9x13 glass or ceramic pan, begin to assemble your lasagna. Start by coating the bottom of the pan with one third of the sauce. Next add one row of noodles, and top with more sauce, a thick layer of spinach, and half of your walnut and nutritional yeast supply. Begin again with a new row of noodles, the remaining sauce and another layer of spinach, walnuts and nutritional yeast. Cover and bake in a 400-degree oven for 35–40 minutes. Remove from the oven and allow it to set for 10 minutes before serving. Makes for a great appetizer, side dish or entrée for any cold weather gathering.

Tip: You can certainly use previously frozen or even canned butternut squash to greatly decrease the amount of cooking time. Please be sure the only ingredient on the package or can is "organic butternut squash."

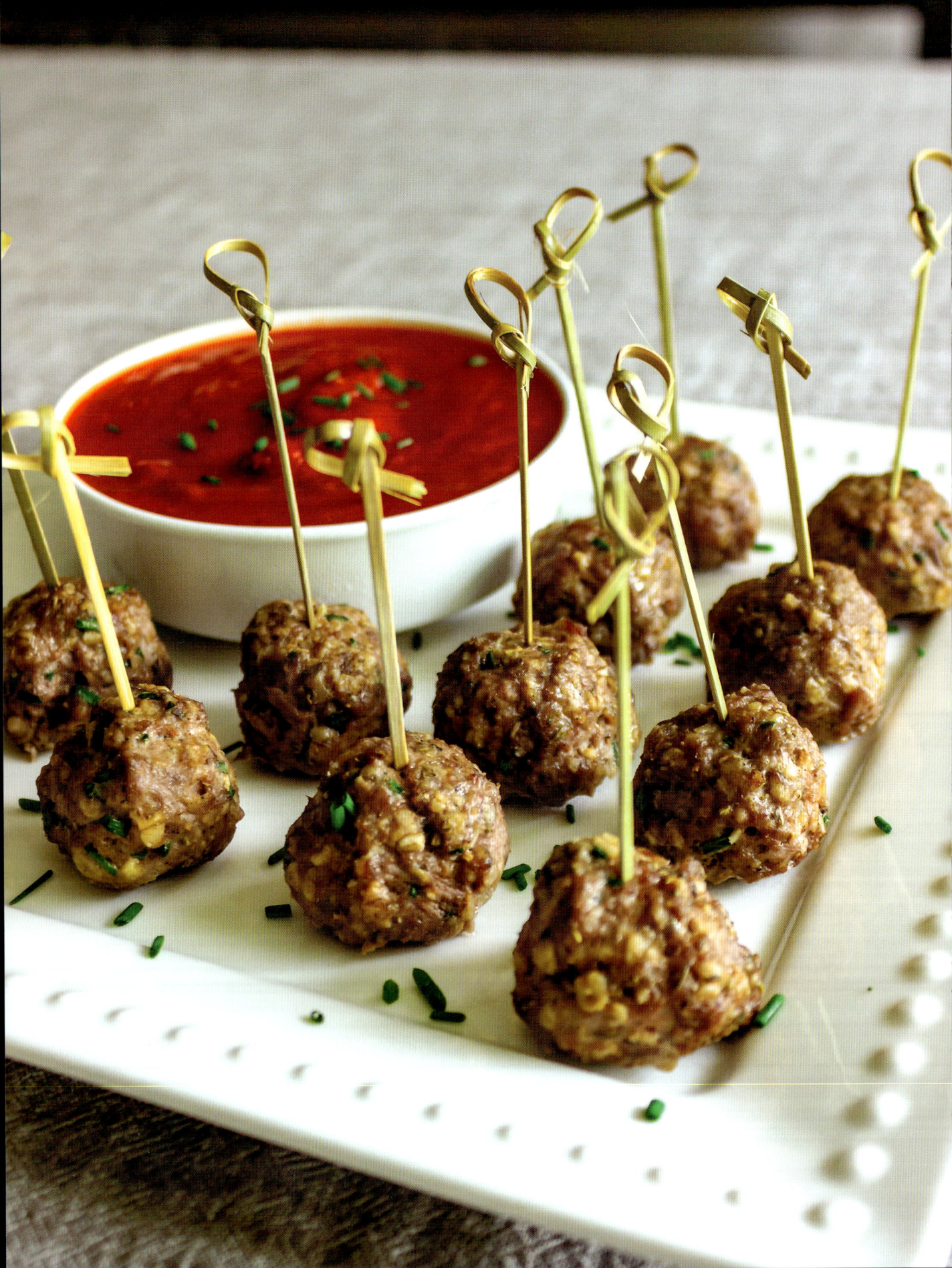

Please Pass the Meatballs

According to my realtor friends, it is the kitchen that sells a home. It is where people gather, celebrate, and of course, dine. Some of my most memorable moments took place with food and loved ones gathered in the kitchen. This recipe is designed to share with others. While these meatballs could certainly be pre-portioned and frozen for individual use, I encourage you to invite over a few close pals and make new memories gathered around your own kitchen.

1 pound ground lamb

1 teaspoon dried rosemary

1 teaspoon dried thyme

1 teaspoon garlic powder

½ teaspoon allspice

¼ cup fresh chives, chopped

1 egg

½ cup nutritional yeast

½ cup oats

Sea salt and black pepper, to taste

Preheat the oven to 400 degrees and line a baking sheet with parchment paper.

Add all ingredients to a large bowl and use clean hands to thoroughly combine. Form the mixture into 1–1 ½ inch balls and place them on your baking sheet. Cook for 16–18 minutes.

Place the meatballs on a paper towel to drain before placing them on your serving platter.

Warm your favorite marinara and serve it alongside the meatballs with some sturdy picks for easy dipping. Open a nice bottle of red and toast to good friends and good food.

Deliciously Holistic: Inspired Favorites

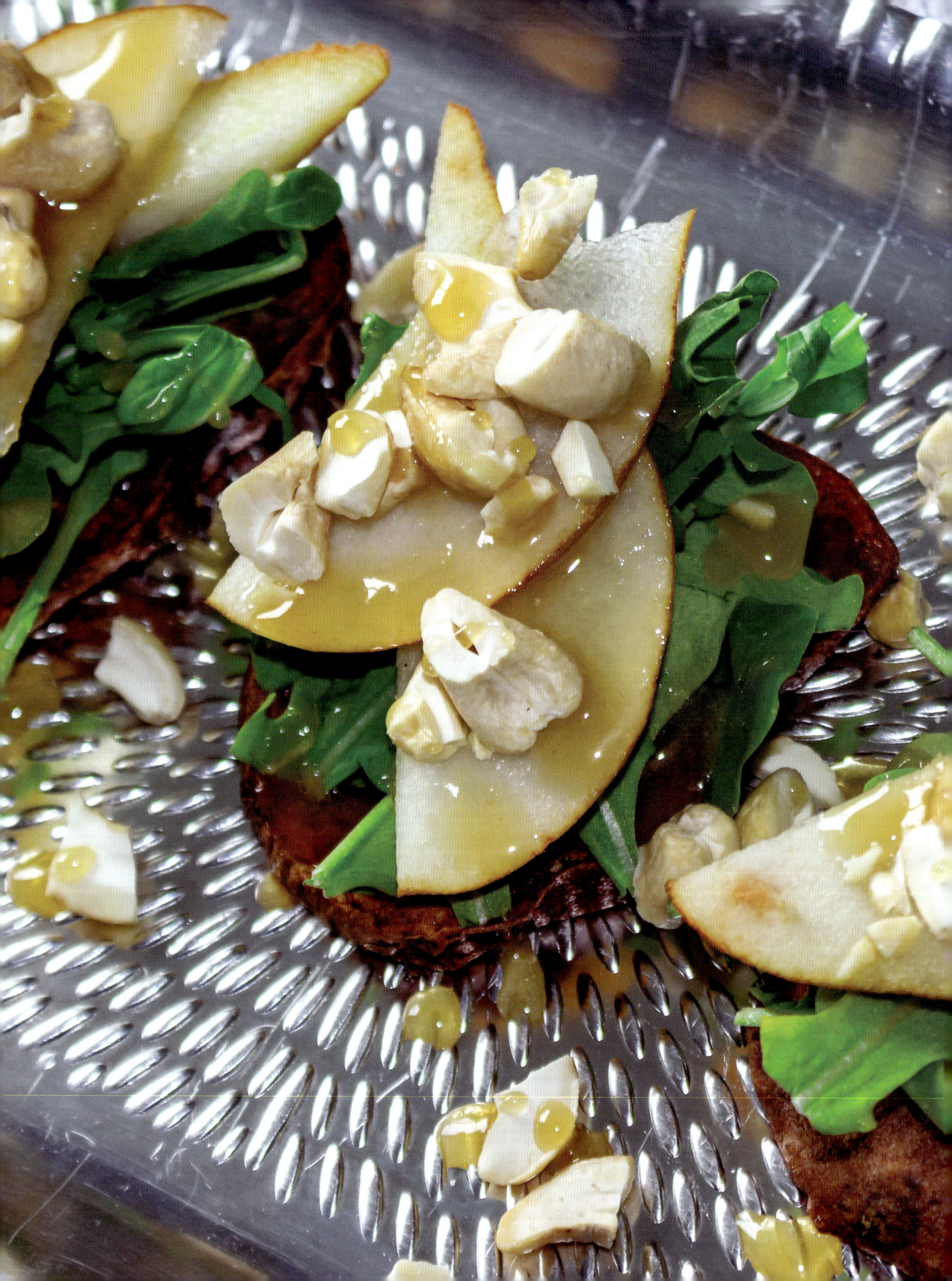

Date Night Sweet Potatoes

Over the years, I have enjoyed many date nights. Like most gals, the anticipation and excitement before the date is half the fun. Now that I'm a married lady in my 40s, I realize it wasn't necessarily the guy I was excited about before every date—it was the food. The best restaurants offered delightful plates of perfectly balanced flavors and colors that left me feeling satisfied but not sluggishly full. When I really started to examine my plate, I realized the food was not complicated, it was simply well composed.

1 medium sweet potato

1 tablespoon avocado oil

1 teaspoon cinnamon

Sea salt and black pepper, to taste

1 ½ cups arugula

1 Bosc pear, thinly sliced

⅓ cup cashews, chopped

¼ cup raw honey

Preheat oven to 375 degrees.

Cut sweet potato into ½–inch slices and place in a bowl. Add avocado oil, cinnamon, sea salt and black pepper. Toss well to coat the both sides of every slice. Lay the slices on a glass or ceramic baking dish lined with parchment paper and cook for ten minutes.

After 10 minutes, remove the potatoes from the oven and flip each slice to brown the other side. Place back into the oven for 10 more minutes until the slices are fork tender. Remove from the oven and arrange the sweet potatoes on a plate. Begin piling a generous amount of arugula on each slice, followed by a few slices of pear and then chopped cashews.

Finish with a very light drizzle of raw honey. If your honey is a little too solid for drizzling, simply warm it slightly on the stovetop to make it easily pourable.

When treating your sweetheart at home with these perfectly composed sweet potatoes, make sure to pair it with a light and lovely cocktail and some mood music. I recommend listening to a little John Legend if you are hoping for a slow dance.

Deliciously Holistic: Inspired Favorites

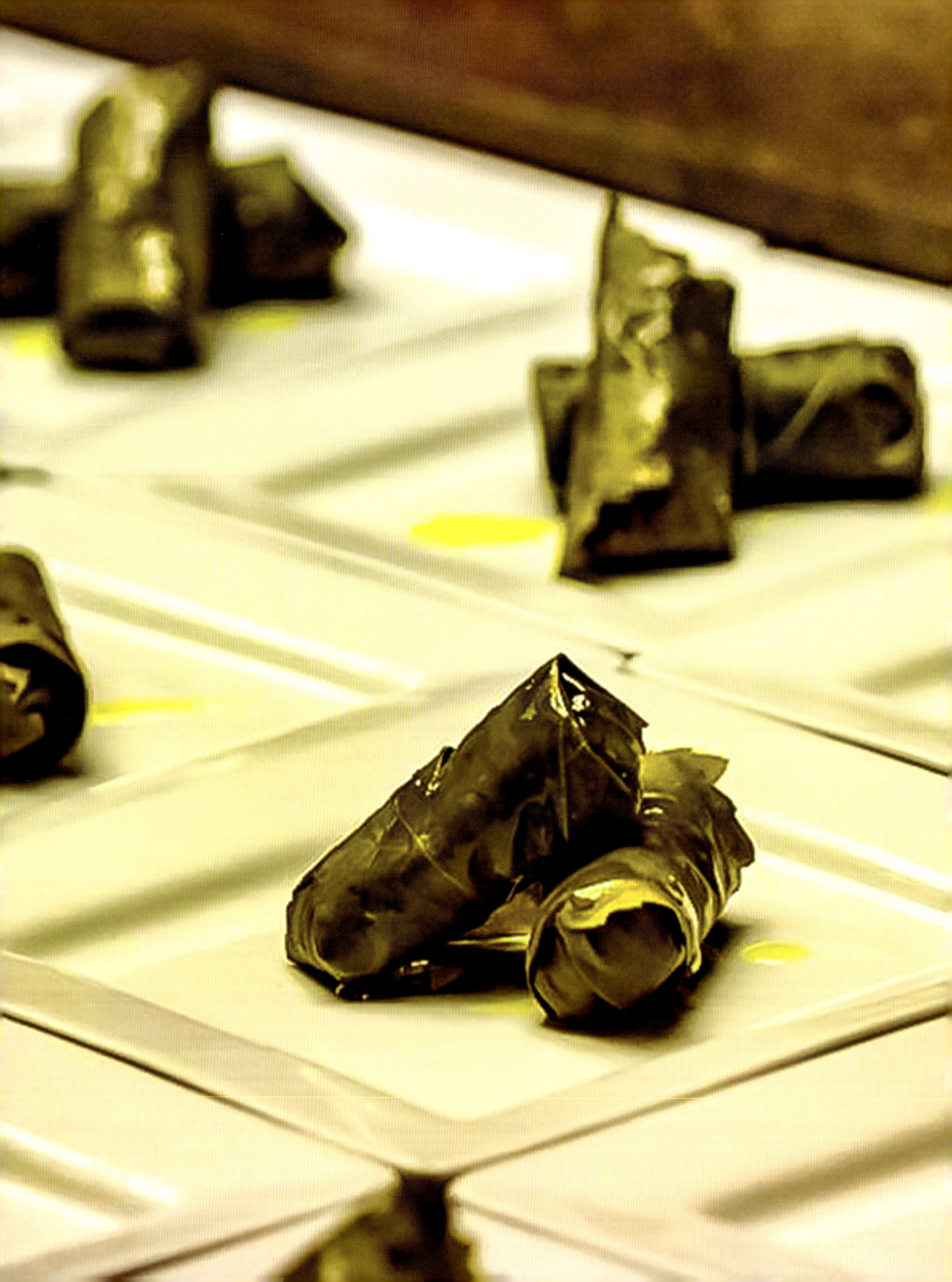

Not my Grandma's Grape Leaves

The most nutrient dense and flavorful food from my childhood came from my Grandma Bette's kitchen. As a child, I believed Sunday afternoons with my grandparents was a time to be on my best behavior and most careful not to spill. Now I realize they were about so much more. Although this version of her recipe uses chickpeas in place of lamb, the purpose remains the same. Spend time in your kitchen to share goodness with those you love. Thank you, Grandma—it's that lesson that has shaped my purpose and my passion.

½ cup wild sprouted or black rice

1 (15-ounce) can organic chickpeas (garbanzo beans)

1 cup sun-dried tomatoes

1 large garlic clove

1 cup walnuts

½ cup fresh basil

½ cup fresh parsley

¼ cup olive oil

Sea salt and black pepper, to taste

Juice of 1 lemon

1 jar of grape leaves (found near the olives and pickles at your grocery store)

Make rice according to instructions on the package and set aside.

Using a food processor, pulse together the chickpeas, sun-dried tomatoes, garlic, walnuts, basil, parsley, olive oil and some sea salt and black pepper. Be careful not to over blend as you want the mix to retain some texture.

In a large bowl, add the mix along with the rice and lemon juice and stir with a fork to combine. Give it a taste test and add more sea salt and black pepper if necessary. Place one grape leaf on a flat surface then add a heaping tablespoon of the mix onto the base of the leaf. Fold in the edges and roll up. Place on a plate or pretty baking dish. Repeat until all blended ingredients are gone.

Store in the refrigerator and serve cold or at room temperature with extra lemon, olive oil and some garlic paste or baba ganoush for dipping. Makes for a great snack or appetizer.

Deliciously Holistic: Inspired Favorites

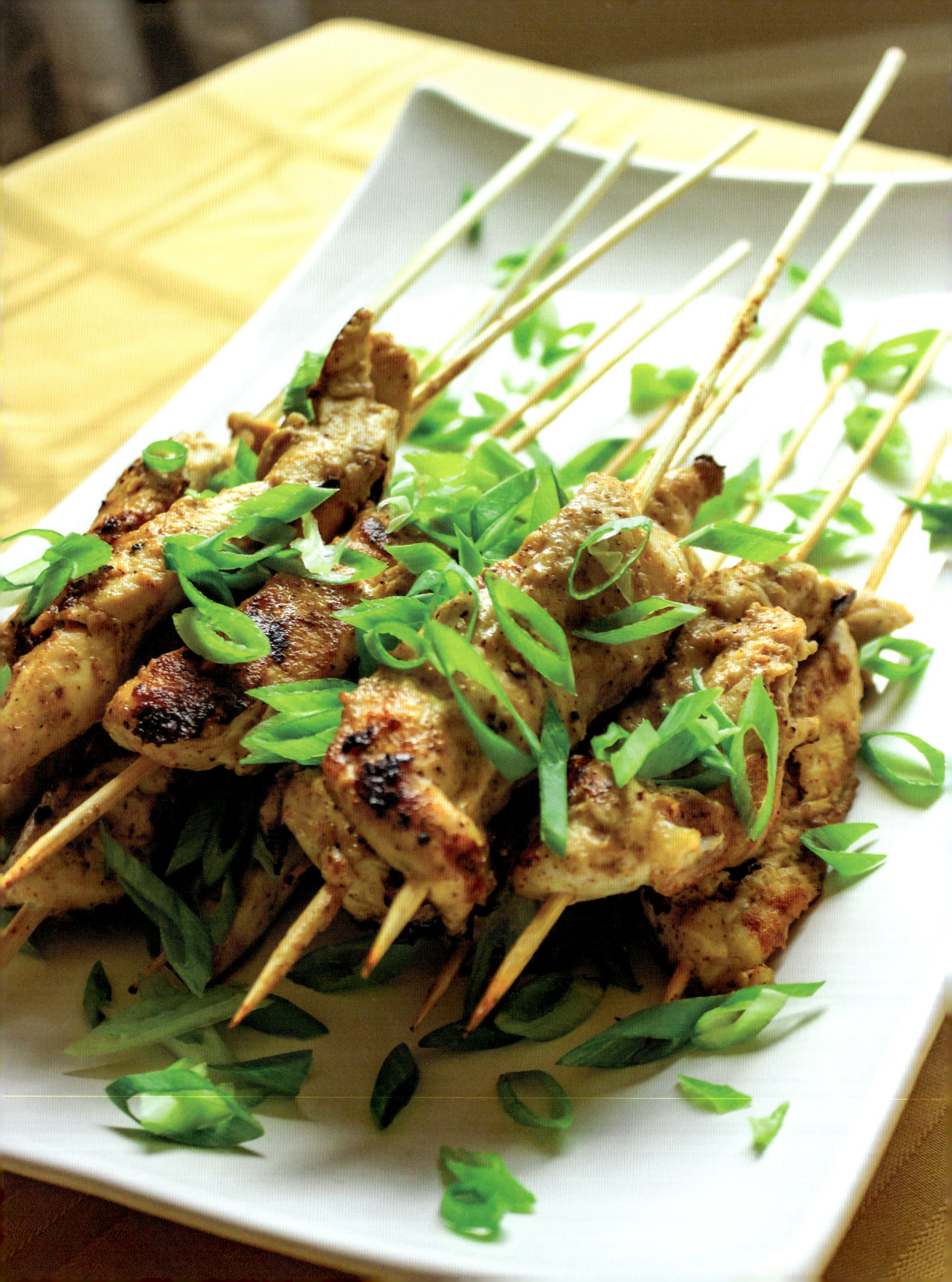

Chicken Satay for your Partay

Food and friends are the perfect combination. I am the kind of gal who finds any reason to celebrate both on a regular basis. And although I can put together a stunning vegetable platter like no other, the party is not complete without a bit of…well…meat. While I'm not suggesting that everyone needs to eat meat daily, you should always consider what your guests will be hoping for when they walk through the door. My own friends, for example, are happy to embrace the inevitable veggies as long as it has an accompaniment fit for a carnivore. This recipe satisfies both the nutrition snob and the meat lover at the party (Both of those are me, of course.).

2 pounds organic chicken breast tenders or chicken breast cut into 1-inch chunks

1 teaspoon coconut oil

1 cup green onion, chopped

Marinade

2 tablespoons almond butter

1 tablespoon tamari or liquid aminos *(gluten-free soy sauce)*

1 tablespoon green curry paste *(use red curry paste if you think your guests can handle more heat)*

½ cup coconut milk

1 tablespoon freshly squeezed orange juice

Sea salt and black pepper, to taste

Place chicken in a glass or ceramic dish and set aside. Next, in a small bowl, whisk together all of the marinade ingredients until they are well blended. Pour the mixture over the chicken and toss well to coat.

Place in the refrigerator for a minimum of one hour or up to 8 hours to marinate.

Melt coconut oil over medium heat in a large cast iron skillet or grill pan. Place 1 tender *(or 2–3 chunks)* on a wooden skewer leaving plenty of space at the opposite end to be used as a handle. Continue the process until all of the chicken is on a skewer.

Add the skewers to the hot pan, and cook for 10–12 minutes or until chicken is no longer pink in the center. Rotate the skewers often to prevent burning.

Arrange the skewers on a platter and top with green onion. Expect to have nothing remaining but empty wooden skewers and a room full of satisfied guests.

Deliciously Holistic: Inspired Favorites

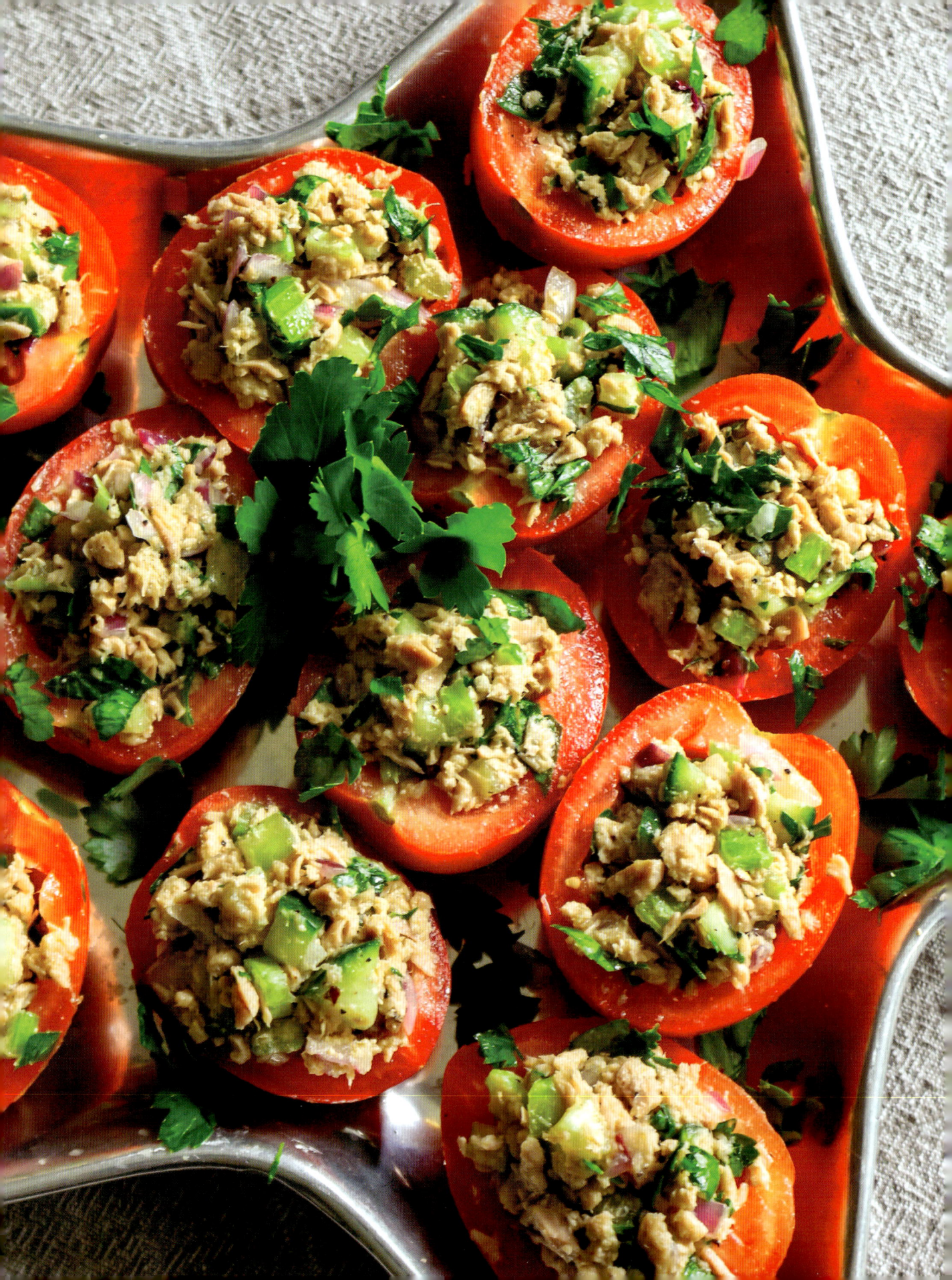

Too Easy Tuna and Tomato Boats

Impromptu gatherings can sometimes turn out to be the very best of gatherings. But figuring out what to serve on the fly can cause unwanted stress in an otherwise live-in-the-moment moment. Having a versatile protein on hand like tuna makes it simple to whip up an elegant but nearly effortless appetizer for your unplanned party people.

6 Roma tomatoes

6 ounces wild-caught tuna, drained (*In this case, the pricier brand is certainly a better product*)

¼ cup red onion, petite diced

⅓ cup celery, petite diced

⅓ cup English (*seedless*) **cucumber, petite diced**

¼ cup fresh parsley, chopped (*plus a little more to garnish with*)

1–2 tablespoons freshly squeezed lemon juice

½ teaspoon garlic powder

1 ½ tablespoons olive oil

Sea salt and black pepper, to taste

Cut your tomatoes lengthwise in half. Scoop out and discard the seeds and place each half skin-side down on a serving platter. If you happen to have a melon baller or grapefruit spoon, either will make this task super simple.

In a large bowl, add the tuna and break up any large pieces with a fork. Add the remaining ingredients and toss well. Scoop the filling into each tomato and garnish with more fresh parsley. Let the party begin!

Deliciously Holistic: Inspired Favorites

Satisfying Snacks & Sweets

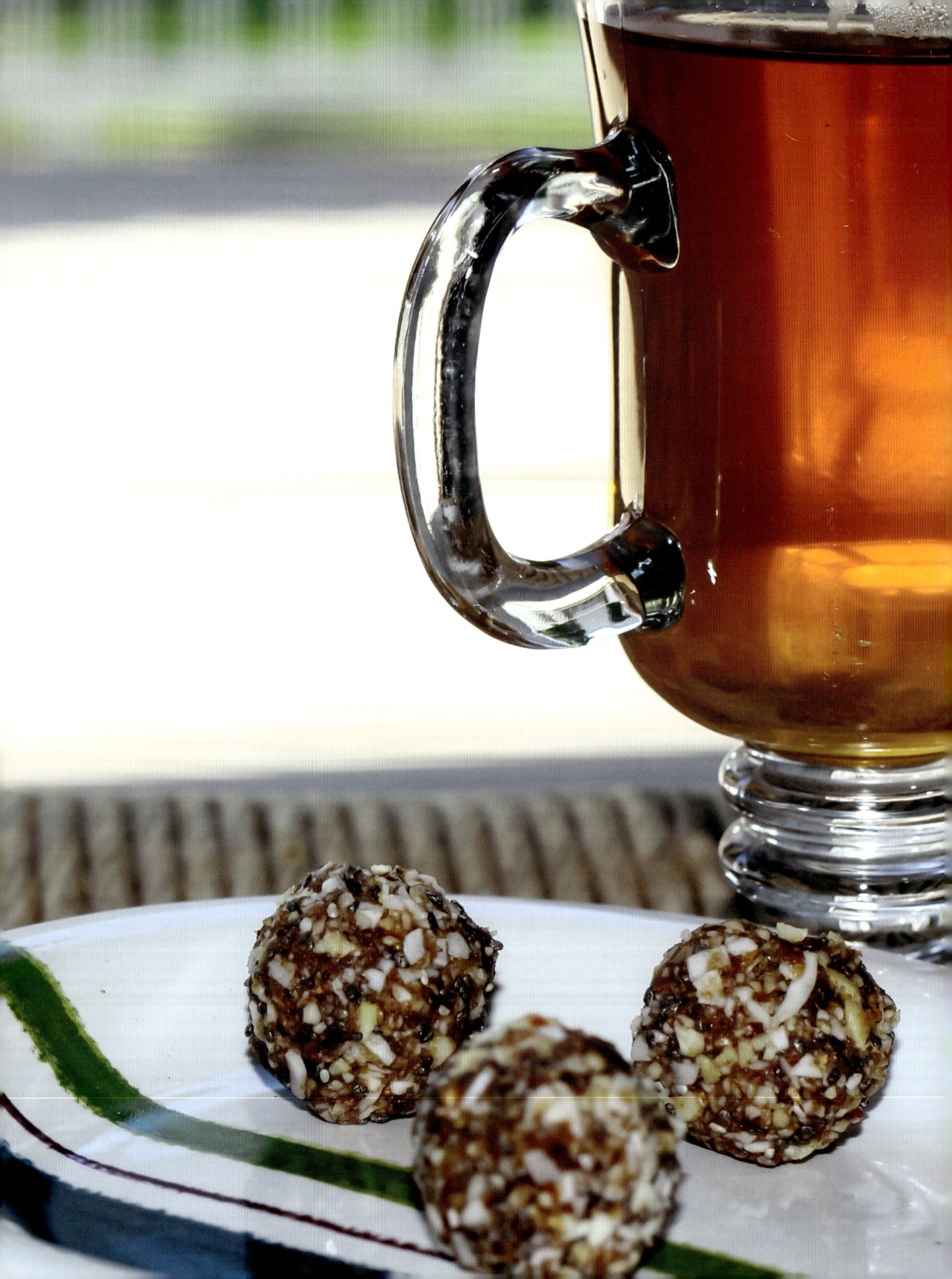

Easy Energy Bites

This snack was inspired by the many moments of hunger that inevitably strike throughout the day when there is simply no time to whip up a batch of muffins or sweet potato fries. These bites are loaded with protein and fiber. Perfect to keep you going until your next healthful meal.

1 cup raw organic unsweetened shredded or flaked coconut

Juice from ½ lime

8 large pitted dates

1 cup almonds

2 tablespoons chia seeds

½ teaspoon ground cinnamon

Sprinkle of sea salt

Blend all ingredients in a food processor until everything begins to stick together. Scrape down the sides to ensure all ingredients are mixed well. Roll into bite sized balls and place on a dish.

Place balls in the freezer for an hour to set. These are perfect to eat right out of the freezer or can be stored in the fridge.

Feel free to play around with the ingredients. Try swapping out the almonds for cashews, walnuts or pecans. Try different seeds as well. You may need to play around with the portions a bit to find the consistency you like.

Enjoy a few energy bites with a cup of tea followed by some deep breathing and a moment of gratitude.

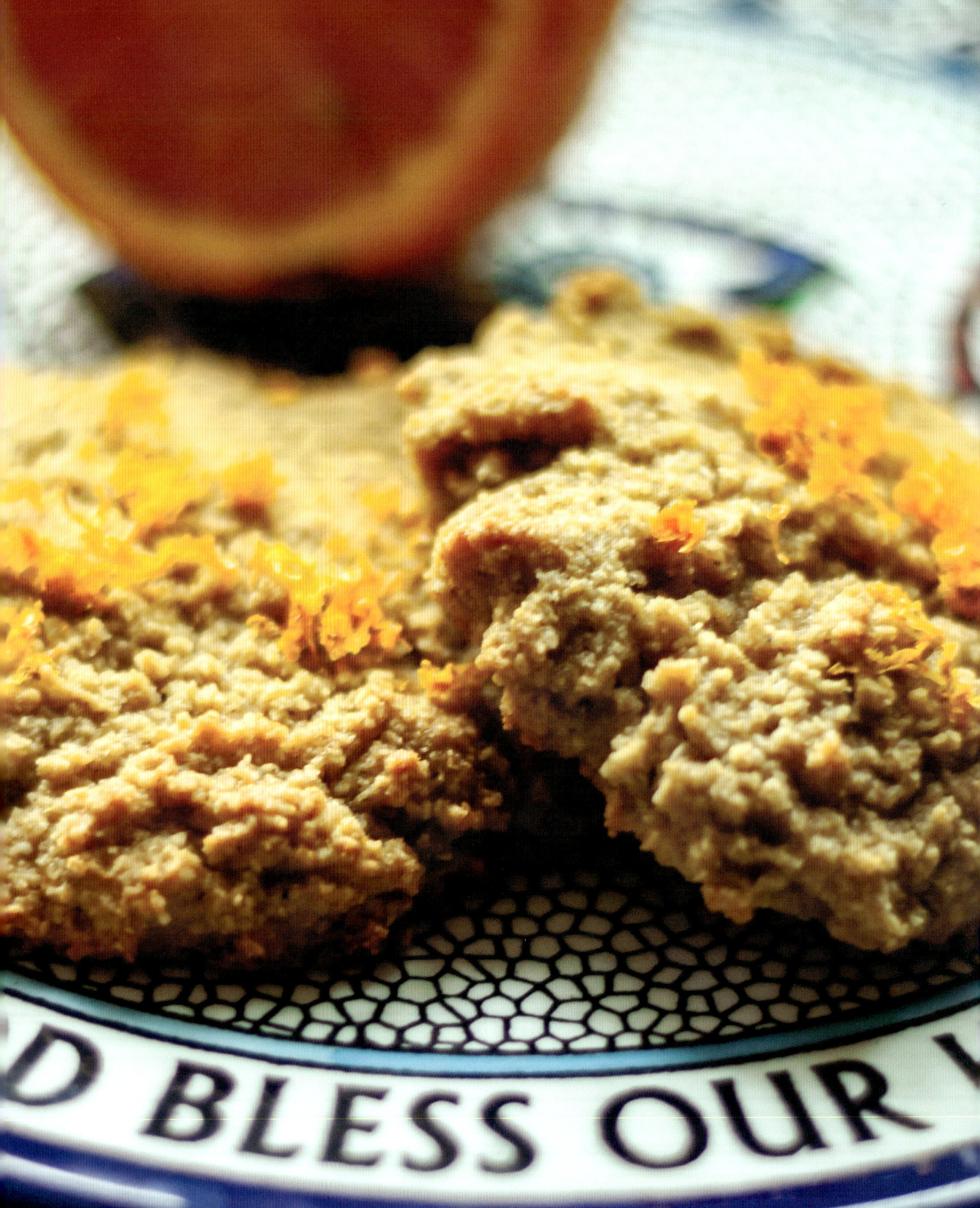

Orange & Spice & Everything Nice Cookies

Everyone has their favorite cookie; most likely stemming from their childhood, a fond memory or a family tradition. If yours is a store-bought favorite, I would suggest you have been missing out on the best part: the experience. The very best cookie is chewy, warm and fresh out of the oven. You simply can't help but to smile after that first bite. These provide every bit of the ideal cookie experience while still nourishing your body. Although they are a delight any time of the year, the combination of citrus and warming spices makes it a perfect holiday treat.

1 cup almond flour

⅓ cup coconut flour

½ teaspoon baking soda

1 ½ teaspoons ginger

1 ½ teaspoons cinnamon

⅛ teaspoon cardamom

¼ teaspoon salt

1 egg

¼ cup avocado oil

¼ cup pure maple syrup

1 teaspoon vanilla

¼ cup freshly squeezed orange juice

Zest from 2 oranges *(this should ideally be organic since you are using the outer skin)*

Line a baking sheet with parchment paper and set aside. Preheat the oven to 350 degrees.

In a medium bowl combine both flours, baking soda, ginger, cinnamon, cardamom, and salt.

In a second bowl add the egg, oil, maple syrup, vanilla, orange juice and half of the orange zest and mix with an electric hand mixer. Add the dry ingredients and mix for 2 minutes. Scrape down the sides with a spatula to ensure all ingredients are well incorporated.

Use an ice cream scoop to portion out 12 cookies on your baking sheet. Using damp finger tips, press down on each cookie. Top each with a bit of the remaining orange zest and place in the oven to cook for ` 9–11 minutes.

Deliver half of the batch to a neighbor in need of a little love. Do not forget to bring a warm cup of coffee and a smile. That is all the ingredients you need for the perfect cookie experience. How nice is that?

Deliciously Holistic: Inspired Favorites | **135**

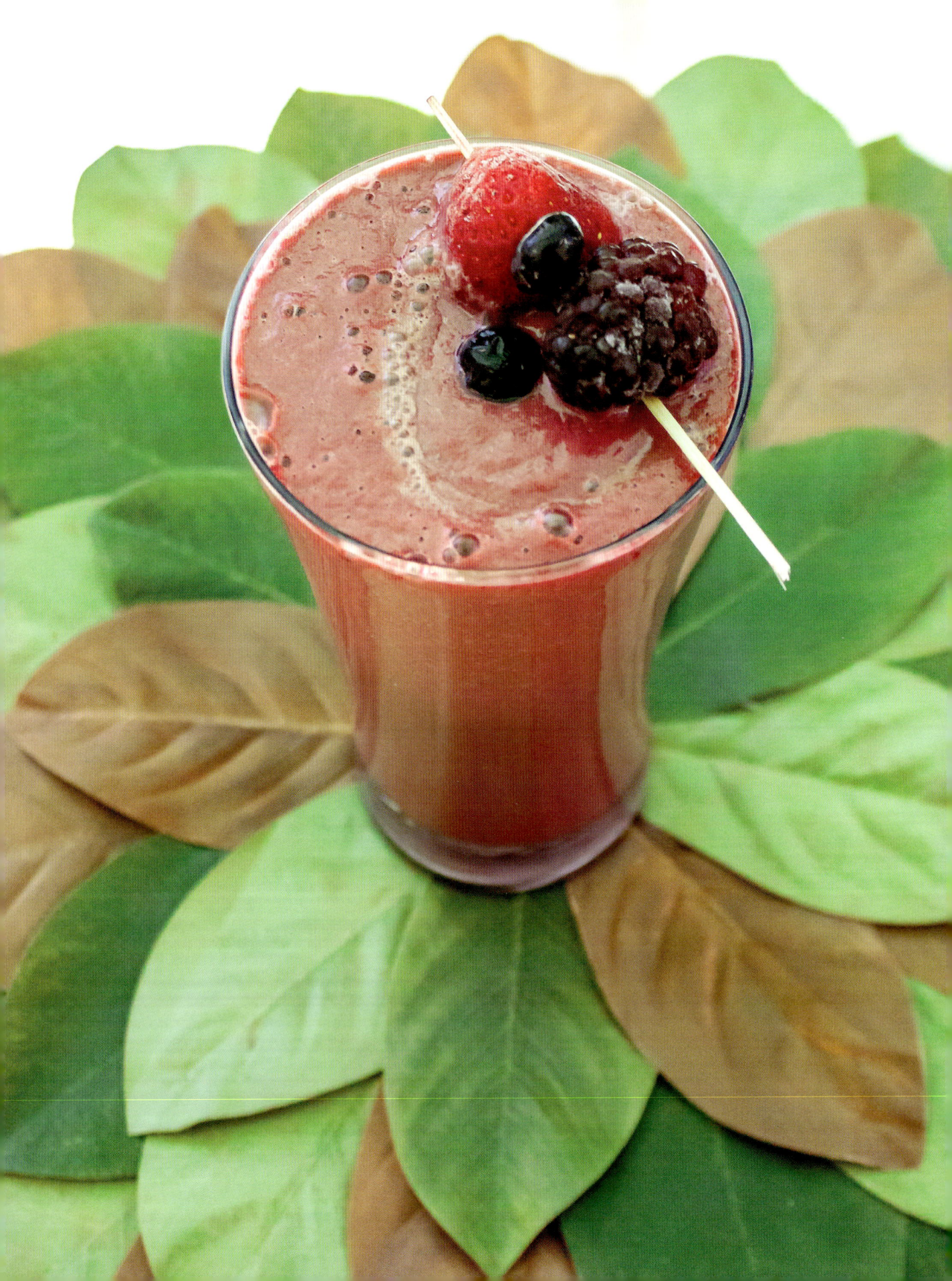

Delicious Daily Smoothie

This one is truly a Holistic Health by Valerie staple. Although I alter the ingredients slightly from client to client based on their particular need or wellness goal, I have found that even after just a week or two of daily smoothies, clients report how much better they feel inside and out. Smoothies are a tremendous way to pack in oodles of necessary nutrition without too much effort. For many of us, our symptoms are related to nutrient deficiencies, so why not start the day by filling your body with the good stuff it's looking for in order to be well? Enjoy this smoothie for breakfast, a midday snack or even as an appetizer while you prepare dinner.

- **1 cup fresh spinach**
- **½ cup cucumber, diced**
- **½ cup celery, chopped**
- **1 unpeeled kiwi** *(yes, I said unpeeled)*
- **½ cup frozen berries**
- **½ small avocado**
- **1 teaspoon raw honey** *(optional)*
- **¼ teaspoon cinnamon**
- **¾ cup unsweetened coconut water or unsweetened non-dairy milk**

Add all ingredients to a blender and combine until you achieve a creamy consistency. You should not be able to pick out a single ingredient in either texture or flavor.

If you prefer your smoothies a little thinner, simply add more liquid and blend again. Enjoy 12–16 ounces daily in a glass or ceramic cup.

Reserve any leftovers for the following day or better yet, hand it to a loved one and encourage them to join you in the clean-eating revolution.

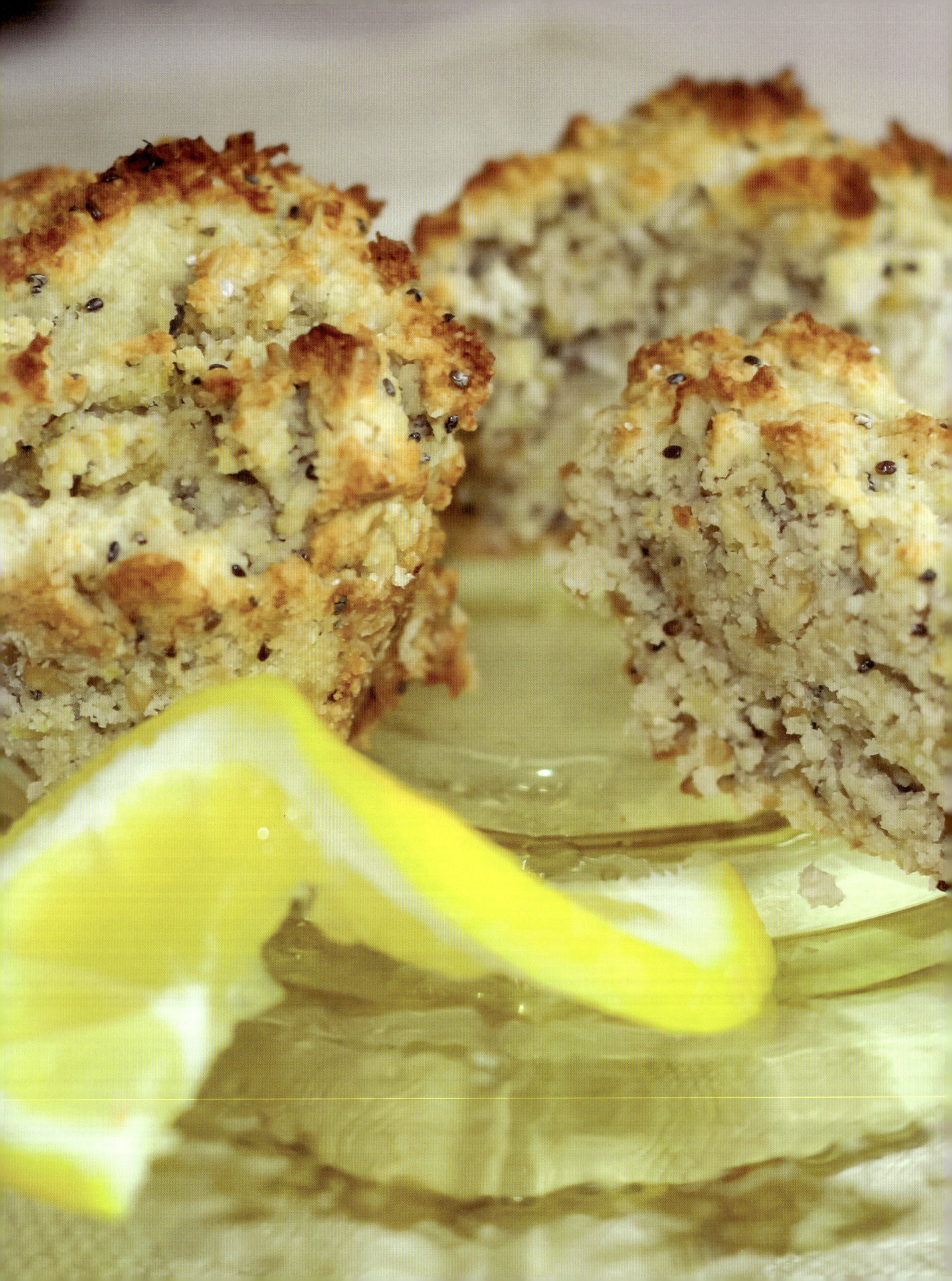

Lovely Lemon Chia Seed Muffins

Chia seeds have quickly become a popular ingredient in the marketing of "healthy" products such as crackers, chips and snack bars. While chia seeds are certainly a super food containing a good amount of protein and a slew of minerals such as calcium and magnesium, one should be cautious about the rest of the ingredients surrounding the chia seeds when reading any label. The easiest way to ensure you are getting a truly health filled treat? Make it yourself. These muffins are loaded with everything your body wants in a snack and you don't have to compromise a thing. Here is a fun tip: wear an apron while baking as it will make for a cute selfie when you inevitably brag over your latest lemony creation.

1 teaspoon of coconut or avocado oil to coat

1 cup almond flour

½ cup coconut flour

½ cup oats

1 tablespoon chia seeds

1 teaspoon baking soda

½ teaspoon aluminum-free baking powder

½ teaspoon sea salt

2 very ripe bananas

⅓ cup pure maple syrup

2 teaspoons organic vanilla extract

⅓ cup avocado oil

Zest and juice from 1 large lemon

Preheat oven to 350 degrees. Lightly coat your muffin pans *(I have both ceramic and cast iron versions)* with either coconut or avocado oil. You can use muffin liners although you will want to make sure they do not contain dyes or have nonstick chemicals in the paper. You don't want any of that nonsense seeping into your beautiful bites of delicious nutrition.

In a medium bowl combine both flours, oats, chia seeds, baking soda, baking powder, and sea salt. In a second bowl, mash the bananas until they are very smooth. Add the rest of the ingredients on the list and whisk to combine. Fold the dry ingredients into the wet ingredients until everything is well incorporated.

Scoop mix into muffin pans. This should make 12 medium-sized muffins so measure accordingly. Bake for 20 minutes or until you can poke it with a toothpick and it comes out clean. Allow to cool before serving to those who have gathered in your kitchen inquiring about the aroma.

Tip: Roll the lemon on the counter before cutting to release more of the juice. Squeeze the lemon over your cupped hand in order to catch the seeds and prevent them from going into your mix.

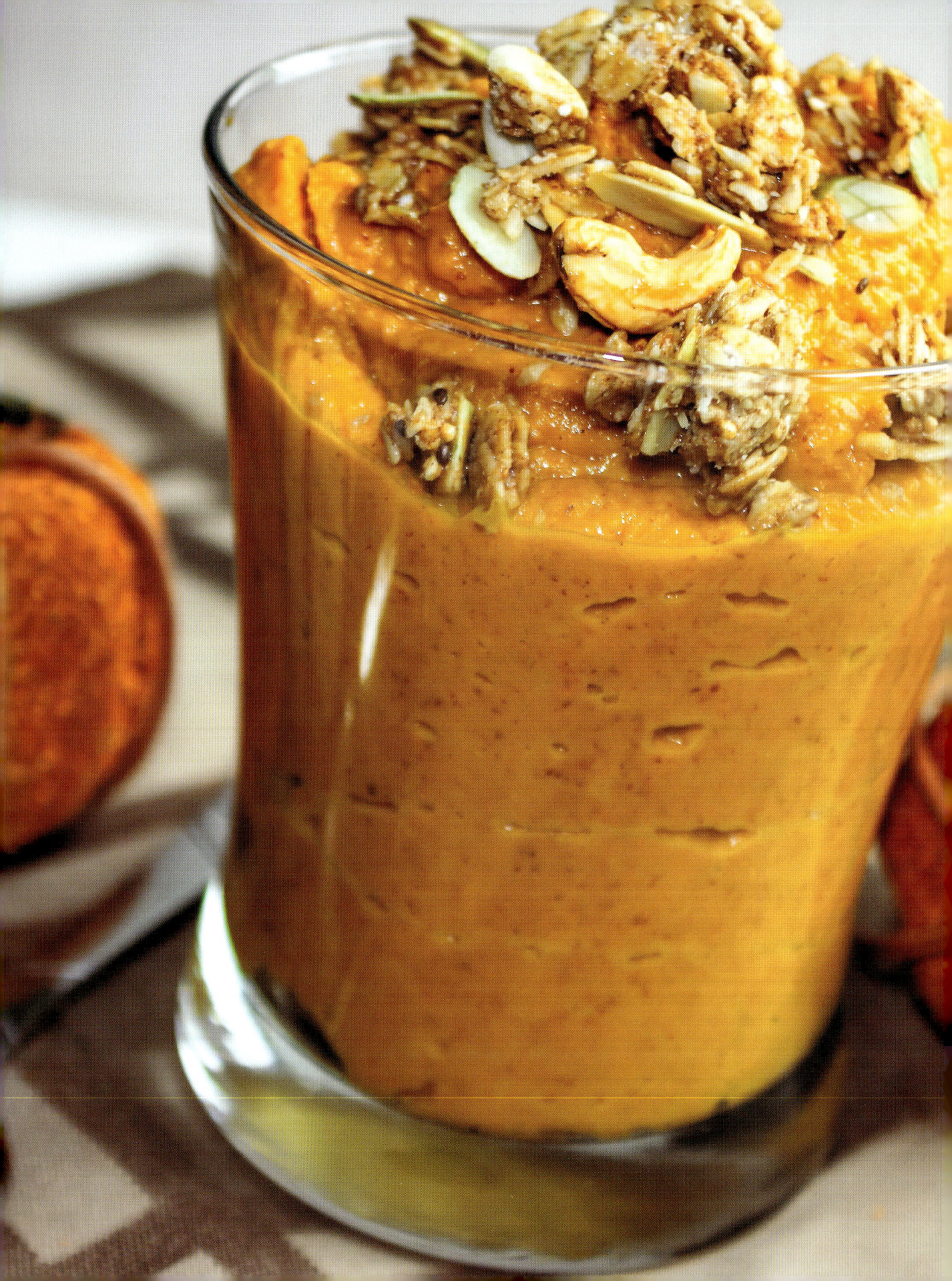

Party Worthy Pumpkin Mousse

Ahh, the fun of fall. The leaves are changing, the temperatures are dropping, and your favorite sweater creeps its way to the front of your closet once again. Although the freshness of spring is a now a distant memory, your kitchen creations can still be a thing of beauty and celebration. This recipe gives you the perfect reason to plan your next party, embracing fall in all of its glory.

- **2 (15-ounce) cans pure organic pumpkin**
- **½ cup canned organic coconut cream** *(if you are opening a new can, use the solid and not the liquid as it has most likely separated)*
- **½ cup organic maple syrup**
- **⅓ cup almond butter with no sugar added**
- **1 teaspoon cinnamon**
- **½ teaspoon nutmeg**
- **¼ teaspoon cardamom**
- **Zest & juice from 1 orange**

In a food processor, combine all ingredients taking the time to scrape down the sides to ensure all components are well blended. Divide the mix evenly between 6-8 bowls, cover and place in the fridge until ready to serve.

For added fun and texture, top with granola, chopped nuts or pumpkin seeds.

Even if it is just a party for one, get out that favorite sweater, find a cozy window seat and celebrate the beauty of fall one spoonful at a time.

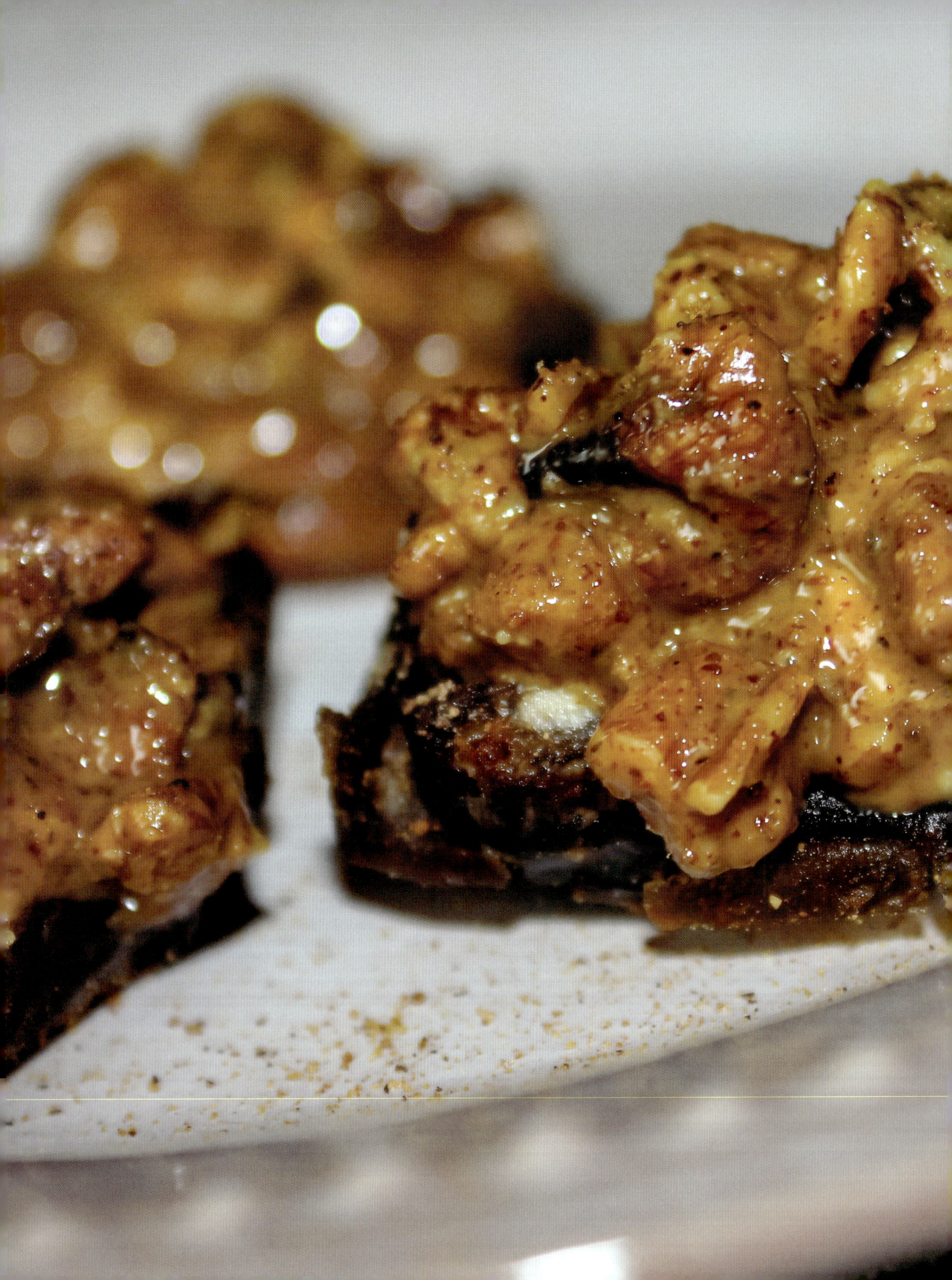

Date Filled Delights

Sweet cravings will happen. Sometimes it is due to a hormonal response happening in the body, while other times a craving is simply triggered by a smell, sight or even a memory. Whatever the reason, these delightful bites are perfect to have on hand when you need a little something sweet. Dates are supremely rich and loaded with fiber so your body will tell you when you have had enough.

- 10 Medjool dates, pitted and cut lengthwise in half
- 2 tablespoons almond or cashew butter with no added sugar
- ½ cup pecans, walnuts, pine nuts, or pistachios, chopped
- ¼ teaspoon cinnamon or nutmeg
- Pinch sea salt

Note: If your nut butter or tree nuts already contain salt—be sure to skip adding salt to your mix.

Tip: *If you need to make these nut-free, simply use a sunflower seed butter and swap the chopped nuts for unsweetened, shredded coconut.*

Once you have each date pitted and cut in half, set them on a plate and prepare the filling. In a medium bowl, add the rest of the ingredients and stir well to combine.

Stuff each date with the mixture and store in the refrigerator. Pairs perfectly with a cup of black coffee and your favorite magazine.

Giving into your craving should always serve as a moment to enjoy something that is just for you—delightful and guilt-free!

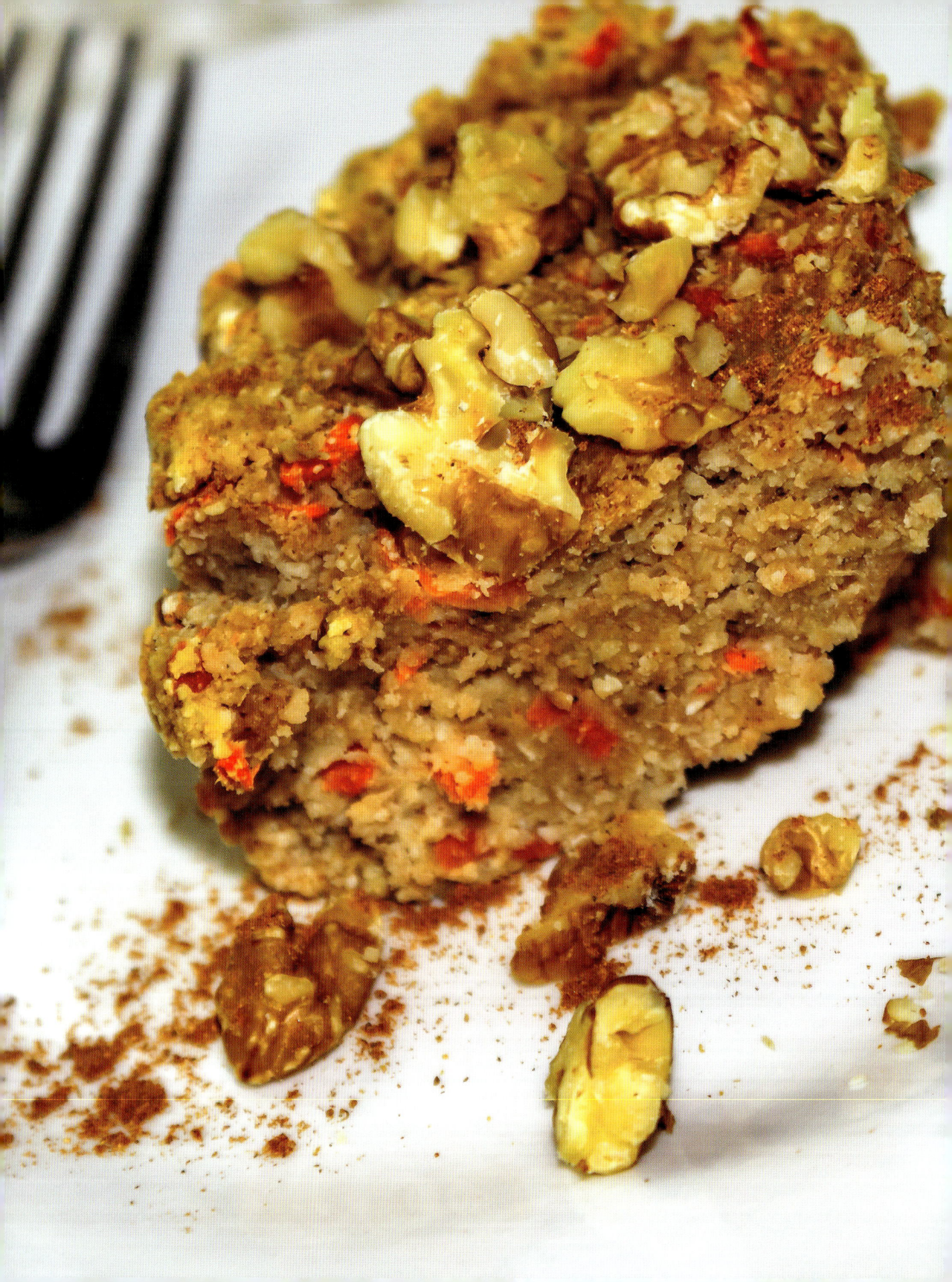

Carrot Cake Inspired Banana Bread

This is one of my favorite dishes to bring to any spring gathering. Typically, I am asked to bring the veggie platter as even my closest friends and family somehow believe I only ever consume raw vegetables. It's more fun to surprise a crowd with this delicious dessert which can actually be served for breakfast as well.

- 3 large very ripe bananas
- 2 eggs
- 2 teaspoons pure vanilla extract
- 3 tablespoons maple syrup
- 1 tablespoon pumpkin pie spice
- 1 cup almond flour
- 1 cup coconut flour
- 1 tablespoon aluminum-free baking powder
- ½ teaspoon sea salt
- 1 cup finely shredded carrot
- ½ cup chopped walnuts

In a large glass or ceramic bowl, mash bananas until they are smooth. Add eggs, vanilla, maple syrup, and pumpkin pie spice and whisk together until well blended.

Next fold in both flours, baking powder and salt until all ingredients are mixed well. Finally stir in the shredded carrot and chopped walnuts.

Place dough into a 9x5 loaf pan lined with parchment paper. Form the dough into the shape of a loaf evenly in the pan. Bake in a pre-heated 350-degree oven for 45 minutes or until the edges are golden brown. Allow to cool before serving.

Enjoy a slice with friends or your favorite book.

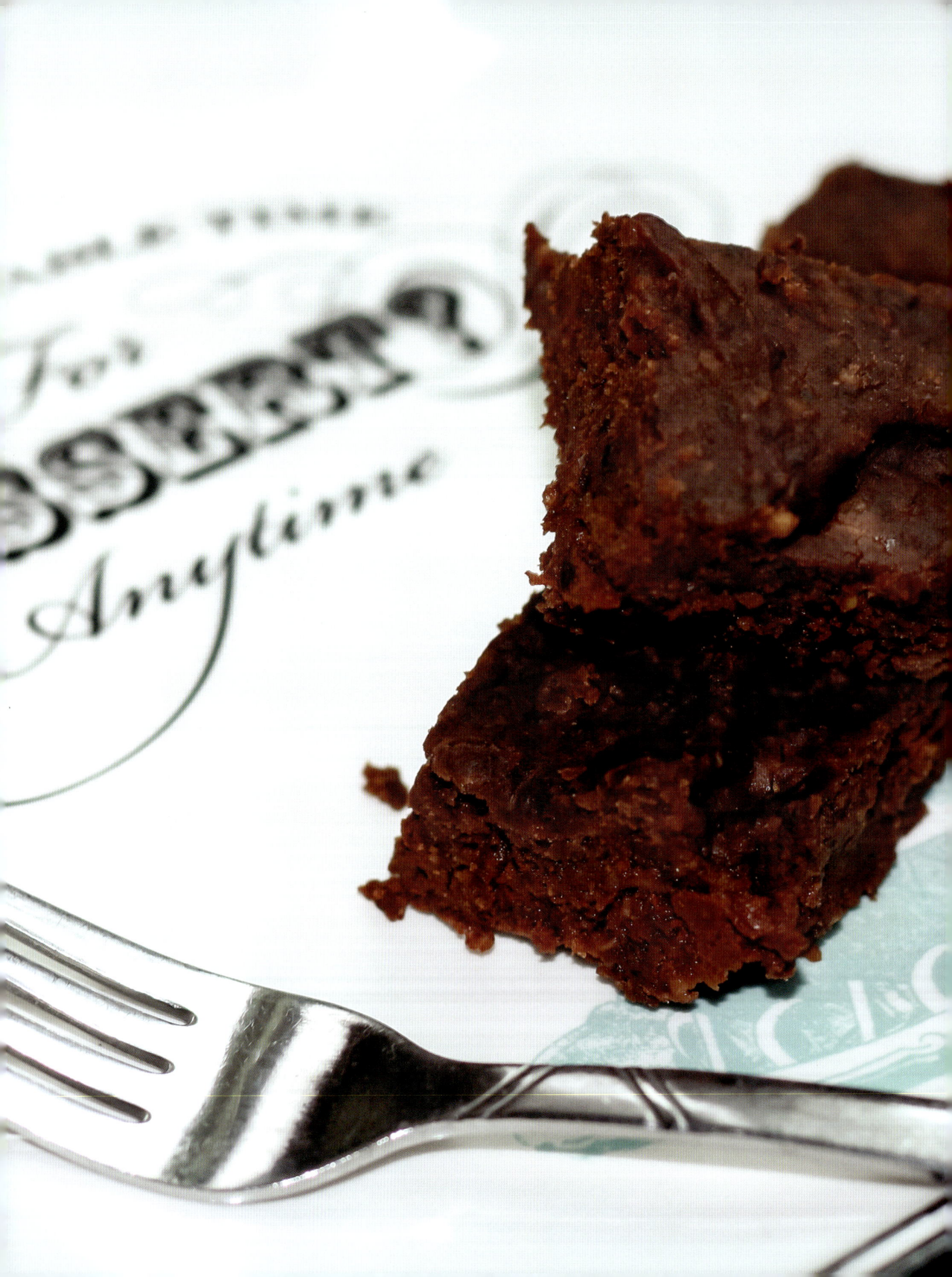

Black Beans in Brownies? Who knew!

Enjoying treats as a child was a common occurrence at our house. In fact, my mother fondly called herself a "chocoholic." As I became a young adult, my own sweet tooth was ever present and tough to deny. At that time, I had a very limited understanding of true nutrition but I did believe that indulging in treats such as brownies would be bad for me and make me fat. Now that I have developed an entire career on the notion that we should be enjoying and celebrating real food—treats are most definitely part of that equation. The earth is loaded with beautiful ingredients that should inspire you to eat well. Discovering they can be scrumptious and sweet is God's little gift to us. Be blessed, my friends and enjoy!

- 1 (15-ounce) can organic black beans, drained and rinsed well
- 2 tablespoons cacao powder *(raw, organic is best)*
- ½ cup quick cooking oats
- ½ teaspoon baking powder
- ¼ teaspoon sea salt
- ⅓ cup pure maple syrup
- ¼ cup avocado oil
- 2 teaspoons pure vanilla extract
- ½ cup non-dairy, unsweetened chocolate chips or cacao nibs

Preheat oven to 350 degrees and line an 8x8 glass or ceramic pan with parchment paper. In a food processor, combine all ingredients except for the chocolate chips. Continue to blend until completely smooth. Stir in the chocolate chips and pour into the pan.

Cook the batter for 15–18 minutes and let cool for at least 10 minutes to allow the brownies to set.

Chocolate was never the enemy. Go ahead— become a proud, self-proclaimed chocoholic.

2019 Health Body, Healthy Mind Expo—Dessert Dash Winner

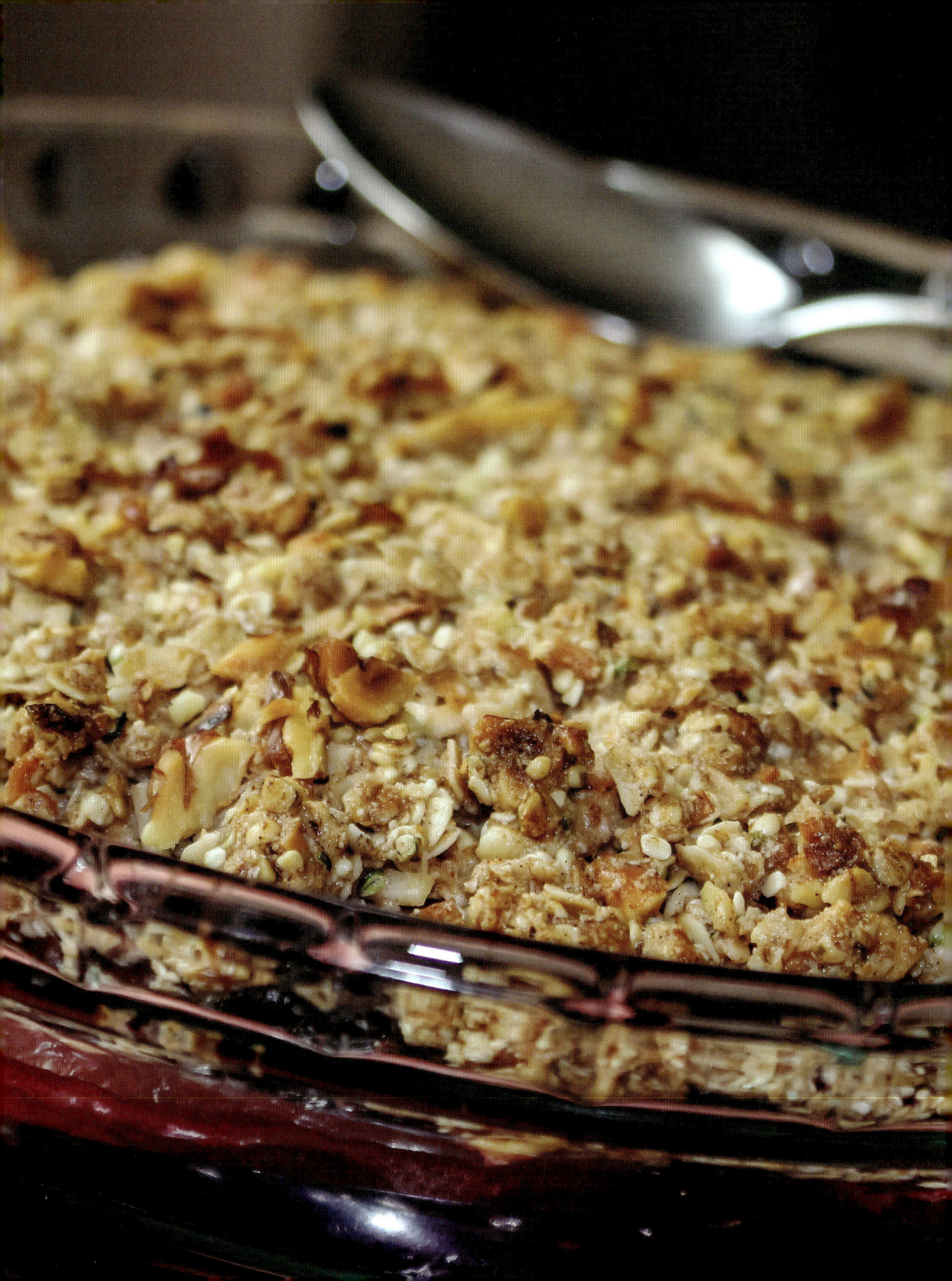

Wonderfully Warming Chocolate Cherry Crumble

A treat, by definition and design, is something that treats our taste buds. But do we have to MIS-treat our bodies in the process? Absolutely not! When most clients first begin to work with me, they assume they will be forced to give up every treat in the house. Soon, they are surprised to learn that I simply want them to eliminate those ingredients that cause harm to the body. After trying a few of my recipes, they begin to understand that a treat doesn't have to equal a mis-treat. This recipe is a perfect example of dessert done right. It is loaded with superfoods and warming spices making it even suitable for breakfast. So, go ahead—treat yourself!

⅔ cup steel cut or old-fashioned oats

⅓ cup almond flour

⅓ cup unsweetened coconut shreds or flakes

¼ cup hemp seed

½ cup walnuts or pecans, chopped

1 teaspoon cinnamon

1 teaspoon ground ginger

1 teaspoon pure maple syrup

1/8 teaspoon sea salt

⅓ cup melted coconut oil (*slightly cooled*)

5 cups organic cherries, pitted (*or a mixture of any dark berries*)

1 teaspoon organic vanilla extract

⅓ cup cacao nibs or organic, non-dairy chocolate chips

Preheat oven to 375 degrees. Place the oats, almond flour, coconut, hemp seed, nuts, cinnamon, ginger, maple syrup and sea salt in a bowl and stir to combine. Add melted coconut oil and mix until you have a crumbled consistency. Set aside.

In a 9-inch glass pan, add cherries, vanilla and chocolate chips. Fold together to combine ingredients and spread evenly throughout the bottom of the pan. Top with crumble mixture and bake uncovered for 25 minutes or until bubbling and golden brown.

Although this is best served warm, I have often eaten leftovers directly out of the fridge and enjoyed it just the same. (*Unapologetically eating from the baking dish, of course.*)

Tip: You can easily substitute frozen cherries if the season does not allow for fresh. Simply place in a glass bowl and thaw in the refrigerator overnight. Pour any cherry juice that remains in the bowl into your morning smoothie or a cup of tea.

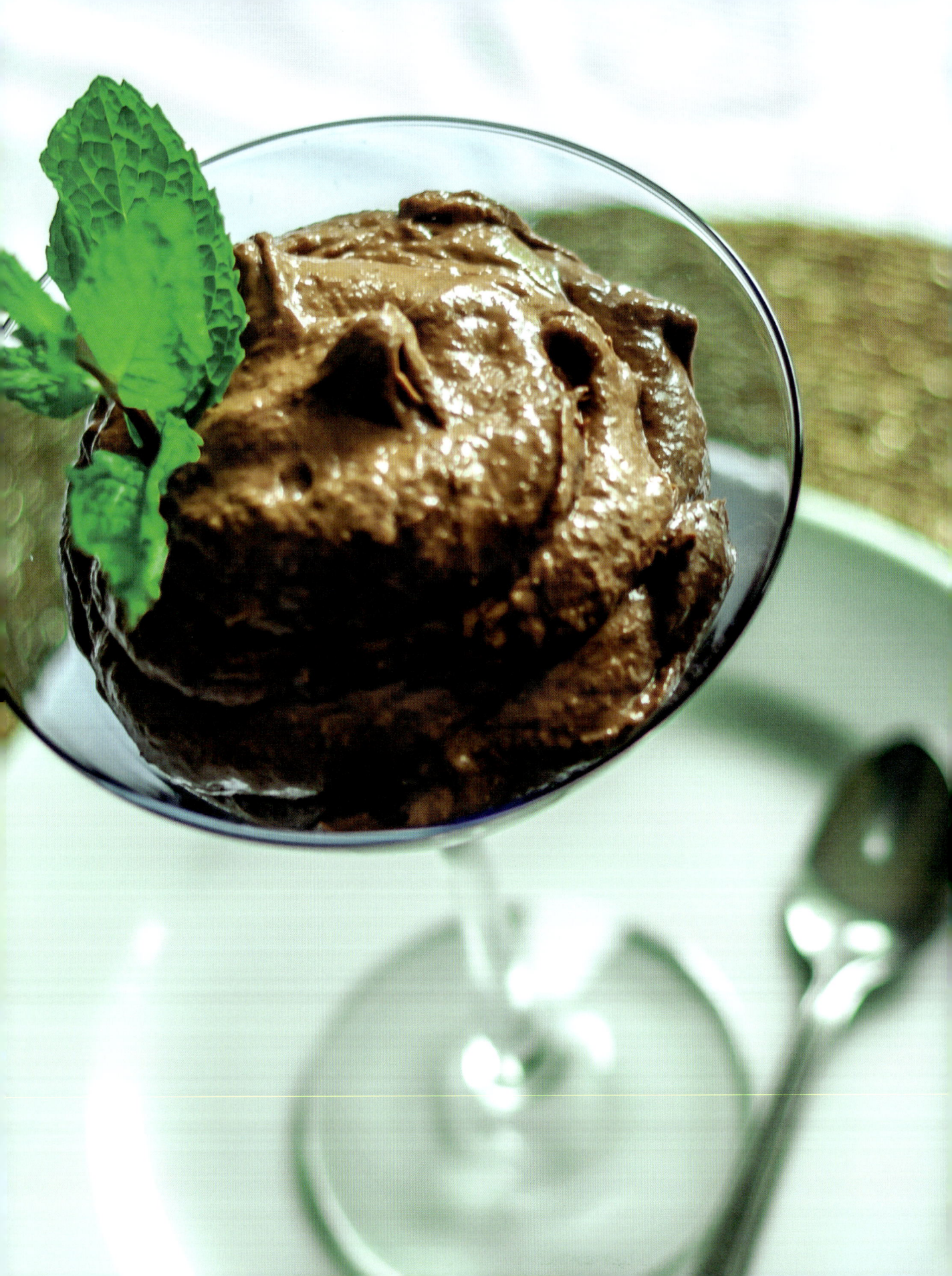

Val's Decadent Chocolate Mousse

In my early days as a nutritional therapist, I only had a pocket full of original recipes to share with my clients. This recipe was by far the most commonly shared among their friends and family. It did not originally include my first name, but since it was passed along by so many that way, I decided to embrace the trend and make it personal. After all, my food is a reflection of my personality: mindful, eclectic, and yes, just a little bit decadent.

2 ripe avocados

4 very ripe bananas

10 Medjool dates, pitted and chopped

½ cup almond, cashew or sunflower seed butter

¼ cup raw organic cacao powder

2 tablespoons unsweetened non-dairy milk

Pinch of sea salt

Scoop the avocado from the peel and discard the pit. Place in a food processor. Add all other ingredients and blend until you reach a beautifully creamy consistency. Scrape down the sides as necessary.

Divide into 6 festive bowls and top with fresh mint or pomegranate seeds.

If the food you put into your body is not already a reflection of your own personality, I encourage you to write down three of your favorite traits then choose your foods based on what will best support the uniqueness of you.

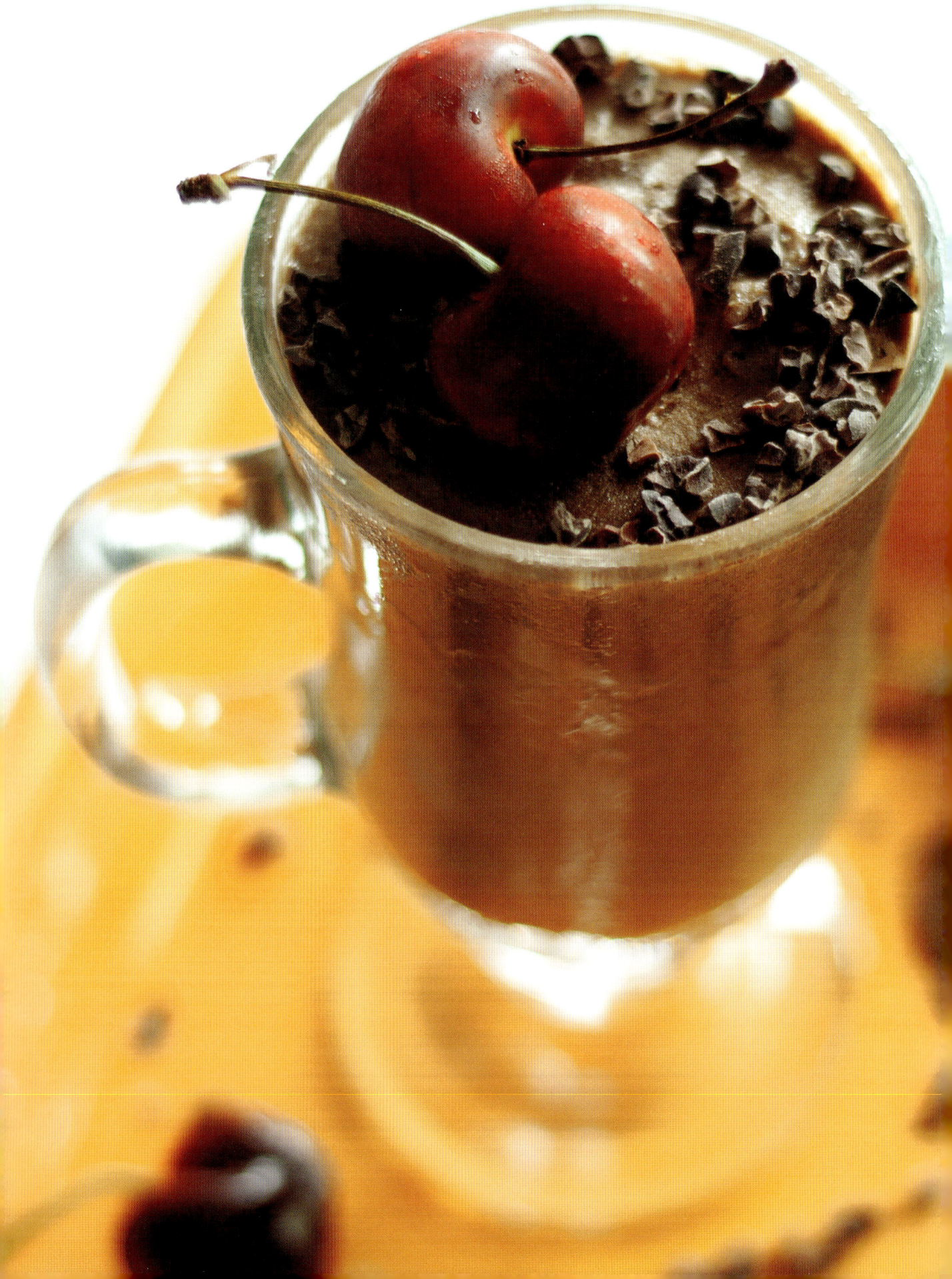

Fun Times Mocha Ice Dream

I have always associated ice cream with the fun moments in life. Sometimes you may get ice cream to celebrate an event or the beginning of summer. Other times you are enjoying it alongside a piece of birthday cake. Whatever the occasion, traditional ice cream is cool, sweet, and of course—fun. Why give up any of it simply because you are following the "Eat Well to Be Well" concept? With this recipe you will never have to.

2 ripe frozen bananas

½ cup coconut cream *(if you are opening a new can, use the solid and not the liquid as it has most likely separated)*

½ cup freshly made espresso or very strong coffee, cooled to at least room temperature

2 tablespoons raw organic cacao powder

½ teaspoon pure vanilla extract

¼ teaspoon cinnamon

⅓ cup cacao nibs

Add bananas to the food processor and blend until very creamy. Add the remaining ingredients except for the cacao nibs and blend again. Stir in the cacao nibs and scoop the mixture into 4 individual dishes, cups or bowls. Cover and place in the freezer.

After completely frozen *(this takes about 2 hours)*, remove from the freezer and allow to thaw slightly for easy scooping. Top with a cherry, of course.

Enjoy this tasty treat while reminiscing over past fun moments or events in your life. Smile. With all of this healthy food in your world, the fun times will keep on coming—one scoop at a time.

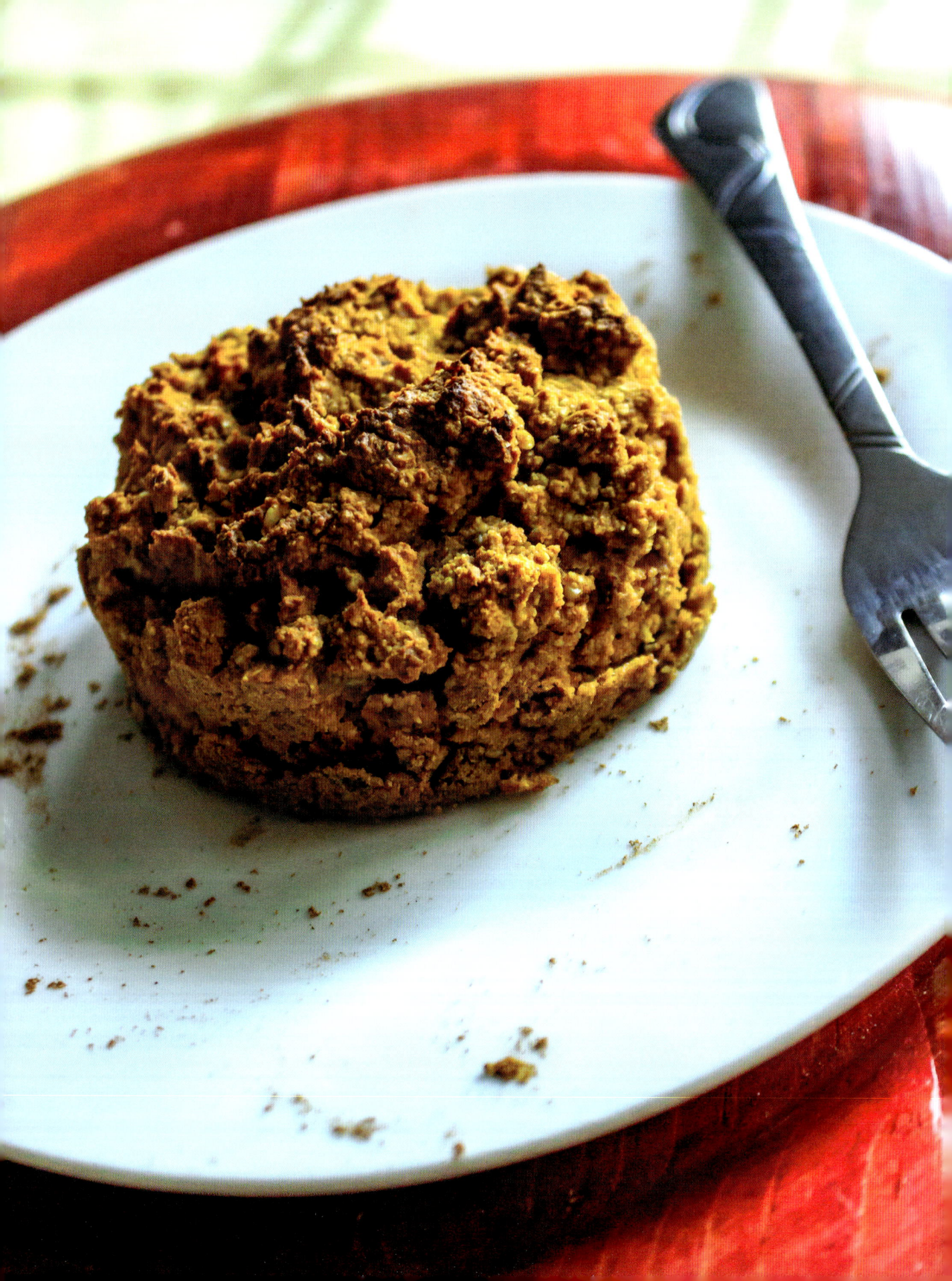

Autumn Inspired Biscuits

Although I treasure every single moment of the summer sunshine, there's something about that first cool evening in September that gets me excited about fall. I am once again willing to turn on the oven and fill my kitchen with the beautiful aromas that come with the new season. This recipe is suitable for breakfast, an afternoon snack, or as an accompaniment to a Roasted Veggie Salad with Warm Maple Pecan Vinaigrette (yes, that recipe is in here too).

1 tablespoon coconut oil

3 cups almond flour

¾ cup steel cut or old-fashioned oats

2 teaspoons baking soda

1 tablespoon pumpkin pie spice

½ teaspoon sea salt

1 *(15-ounce)* **can organic pumpkin or butternut squash**

1 *(5-ounce)* **carton plain, unsweetened non-dairy yogurt**

1 teaspoon organic vanilla extract

1 tablespoon pure maple syrup

Use coconut oil to grease the inside of your ceramic or cast-iron biscuit or muffin baking pans. Preheat oven to 425 degrees.

In a large bowl, add the flour, oats, baking soda, pumpkin pie spice, and sea salt. Use a whisk or fork to combine. Make a small well in the center and add the pumpkin (or squash), yogurt, vanilla, maple syrup and fold into the existing ingredients.

Divide the batter evenly and bake for 25 minutes or until a toothpick comes out clean from the center. Allow to cool in the pan before serving.

Tip: *Typically, biscuit pans are much larger than muffin-sized pans so you may end up with as few as 8 or as many as 12 biscuits depending on the type of baking pan you use.*

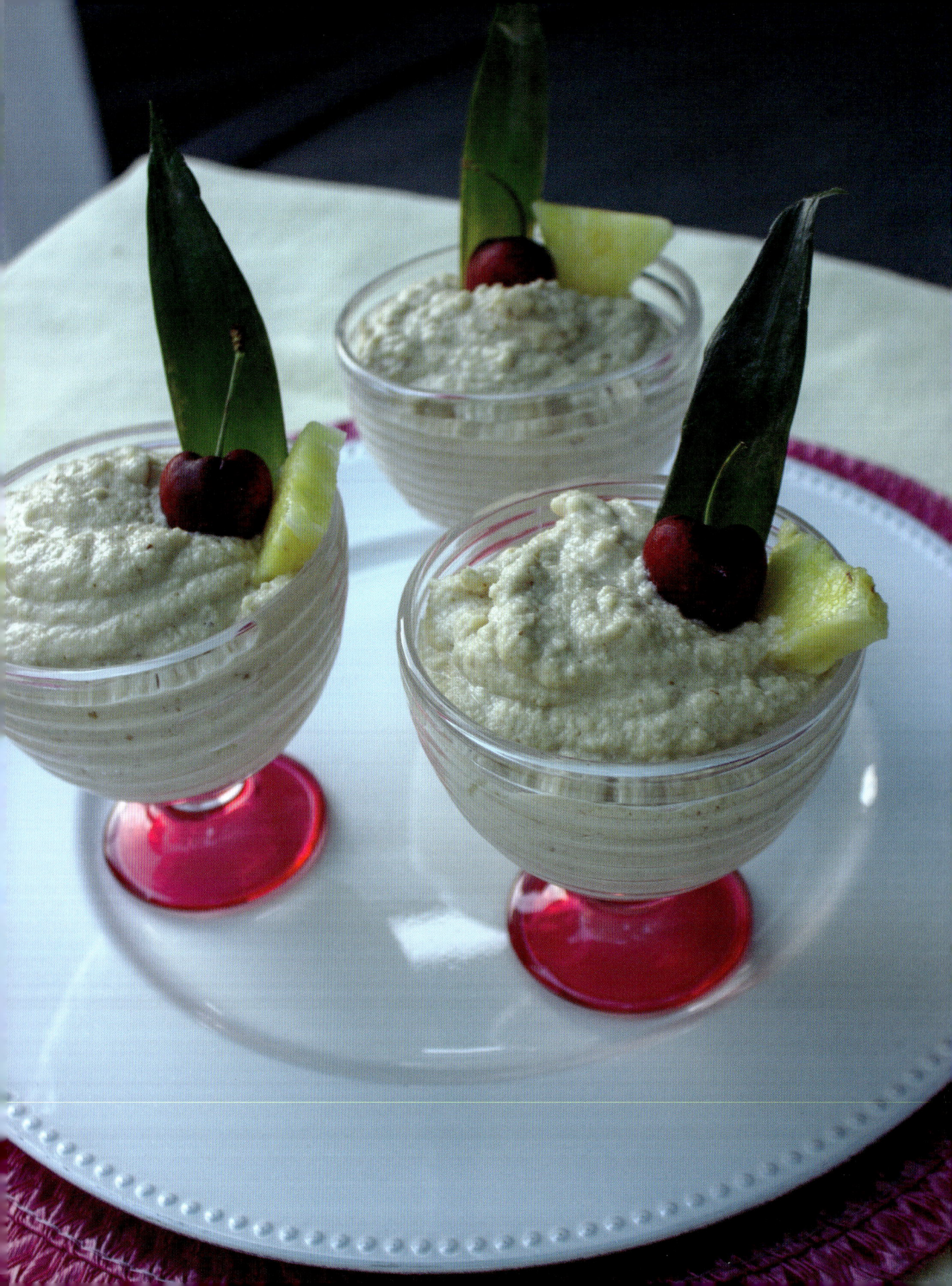

Take Me to Hawaii Please, Pudding

About eight years ago, I was blessed with the opportunity to visit the gorgeous island of Maui. I was able to explore every bit of the island and experienced a complete sensory overload by the stunning natural beauty and island aromas. The food, as you may have guessed, far surpassed anything I had experienced before. Since the fruit is so fresh and plentiful, I truly never felt the need to seek out dessert although it was evident that they were simple, fresh and light. This recipe is a tribute to a truly beautiful place that offers the very best of nature's sweet stuff.

2 cups raw macadamia nuts

8 pitted dates

1 ⅓ cups shredded unsweetened coconut

1 cup unsweetened coconut water

1 cup pineapple juice

¼ teaspoon sea salt

In a food processor, add the dry ingredients then the wet ingredients on top. Blend for at least 2–3 minutes or until you achieve a very creamy consistency. Scrape down the sides as necessary to incorporate all ingredients.

Divide into 4 serving bowls and place in the refrigerator to chill for 15 minutes. Garnish with a piece of pineapple, a cherry and a fun drink umbrella.

It won't quite replace an actual island experience, but it is enough to tide you over until your next trip. Aloha!

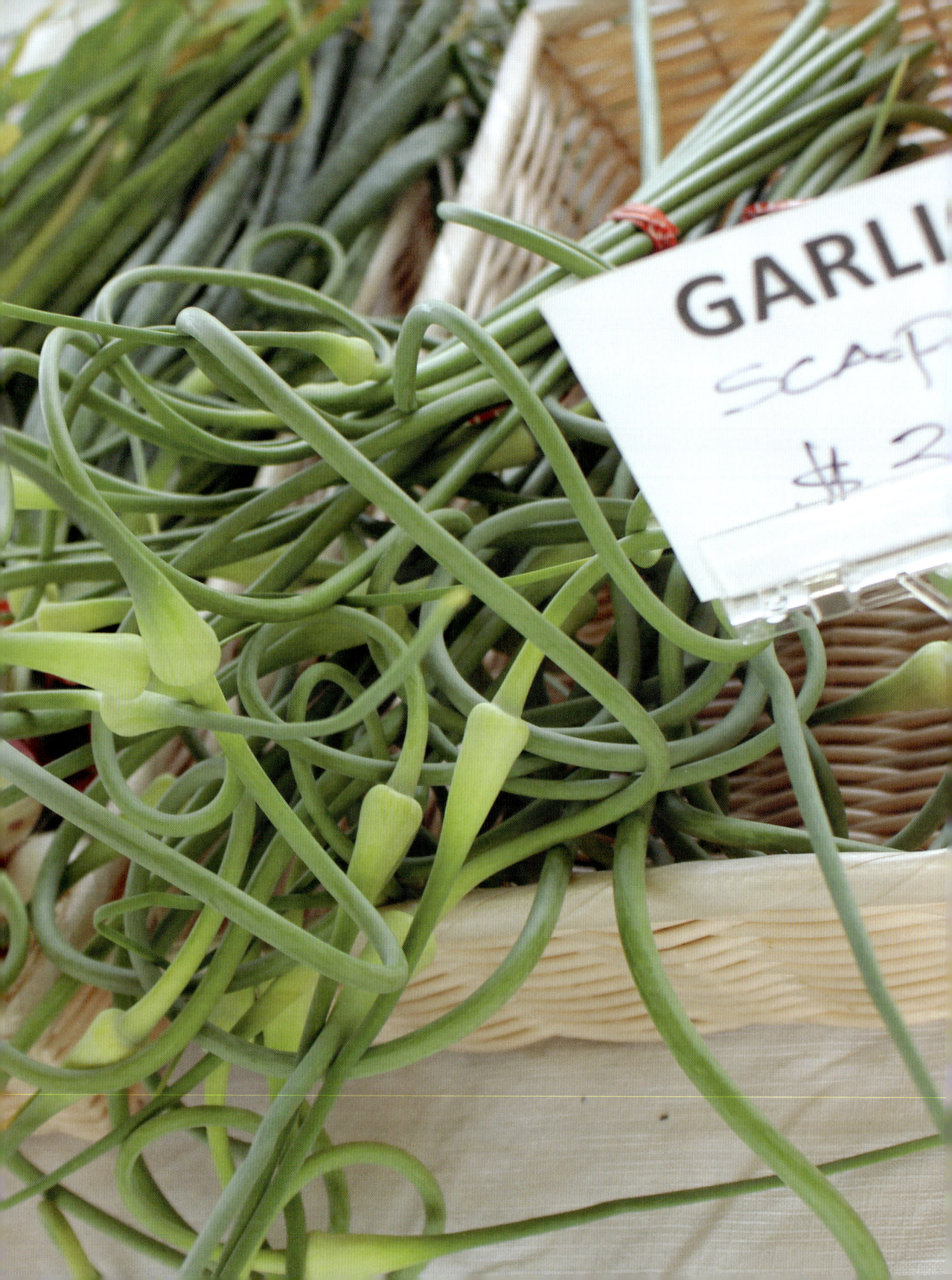

About the Author

Valerie Penz, owner of Holistic Health by Valerie, LLC is a Certified Nutritional Therapist and a holistic wellness advocate. She specializes in teaching others how to find optimal health through the use of proper nutrition, stress reduction, meditation, toxin elimination, and exercise. She works with both children and adults and offers personal counseling, cooking classes, public seminars and corporate wellness programs. You can also find her regularly volunteering her time in support of her community, her church, and any other cause God places on her heart.

Valerie currently lives in Lake Orion, Michigan with her two children, Noah and Ella, and her husband, Brian.

For more information on Holistic Health by Valerie, LLC or to contact Valerie please visit www.holistichealthbyvalerie.com.

Facebook: HHBV nutrition & wellness coaching

Instagram: holistic Valerie

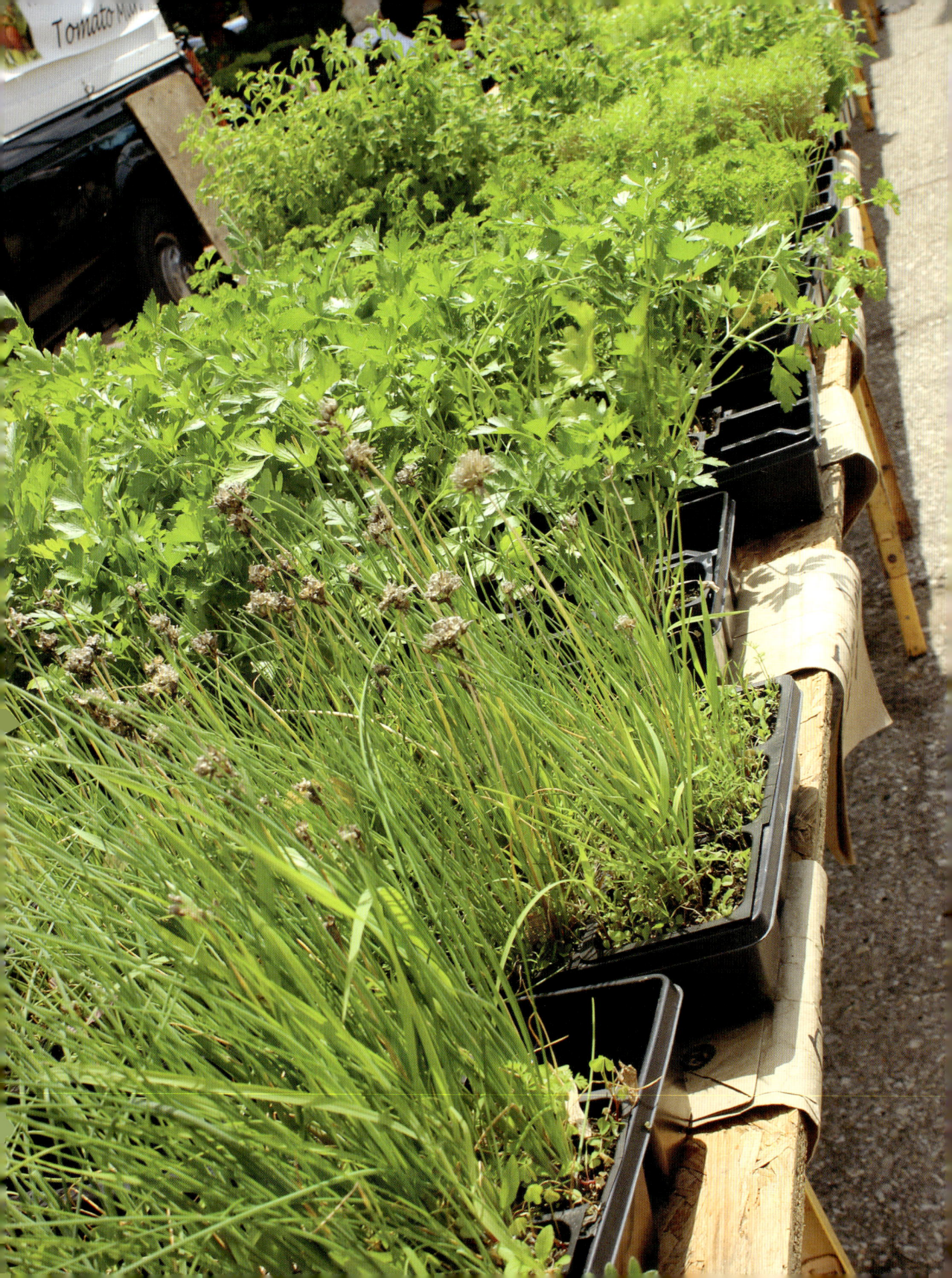

Acknowledgements

First, I must acknowledge my clients, class guests and lecture attendees. So many of you encouraged me to write this book and inspired me with your own success stories in your quest to be well. It gives me so much joy when I receive a picture of a meal you enjoyed based on following one of my recipes. Be proud of every effort and keep on cooking.

Victoria Connolly and Gail Grandy. Without the two of you, I would not have had the opportunity to develop my Deliciously Holistic cooking classes into the fun and fabulous events they are today. You each have unique gifts and talents that allowed me to continue to fill every seat and send every guest home with a happy belly and a smile. Without the class success, this book would still be a hopeful dream for the future. Your support and friendship have meant more than you know and I can't thank you enough.

To the Orion Area Chamber of Commerce and the Orion community. So much of what Holistic Health by Valerie has grown into today I attribute to the people and opportunities afforded by this community. I thank you for your years of support and willingness to try something new. I am so proud to call Lake Orion my home. Go Dragons!

My very talented *Deliciously Holistic—Inspired Favorites* team. I can't thank you all enough for your hard work and dedication to this project. I am so grateful for each of you; your patience, your expertise and most importantly your friendship are the reasons these recipes have made their way from countless notepads to a publication worthy of pride.

My fellow wellness-minded friends and colleagues. Thank you for being another source of inspiration, reference and guidance to all those who seek holistic living. We may have different offices, modalities and talents, but the reason we do what we do is the same. We all understand that true health does not come from a pill, shake, patch or other manufactured product. It is the combination of caring for the mind, body and spirit in a way that was intended by nature and our Creator. Thank you all for being unwavering in a world looking for a quick fix.

To my husband, children and my dearest friends. Each one of you are part of this story. You inspire me daily to create new recipes worthy of serving to you. The secret ingredient is always love; thank you for keeping my heart full and my soul motivated for more.

Finally, and most importantly, I thank God. It is only by His grace that my path has led me to this. It is truly His story. I just get to be the messenger.

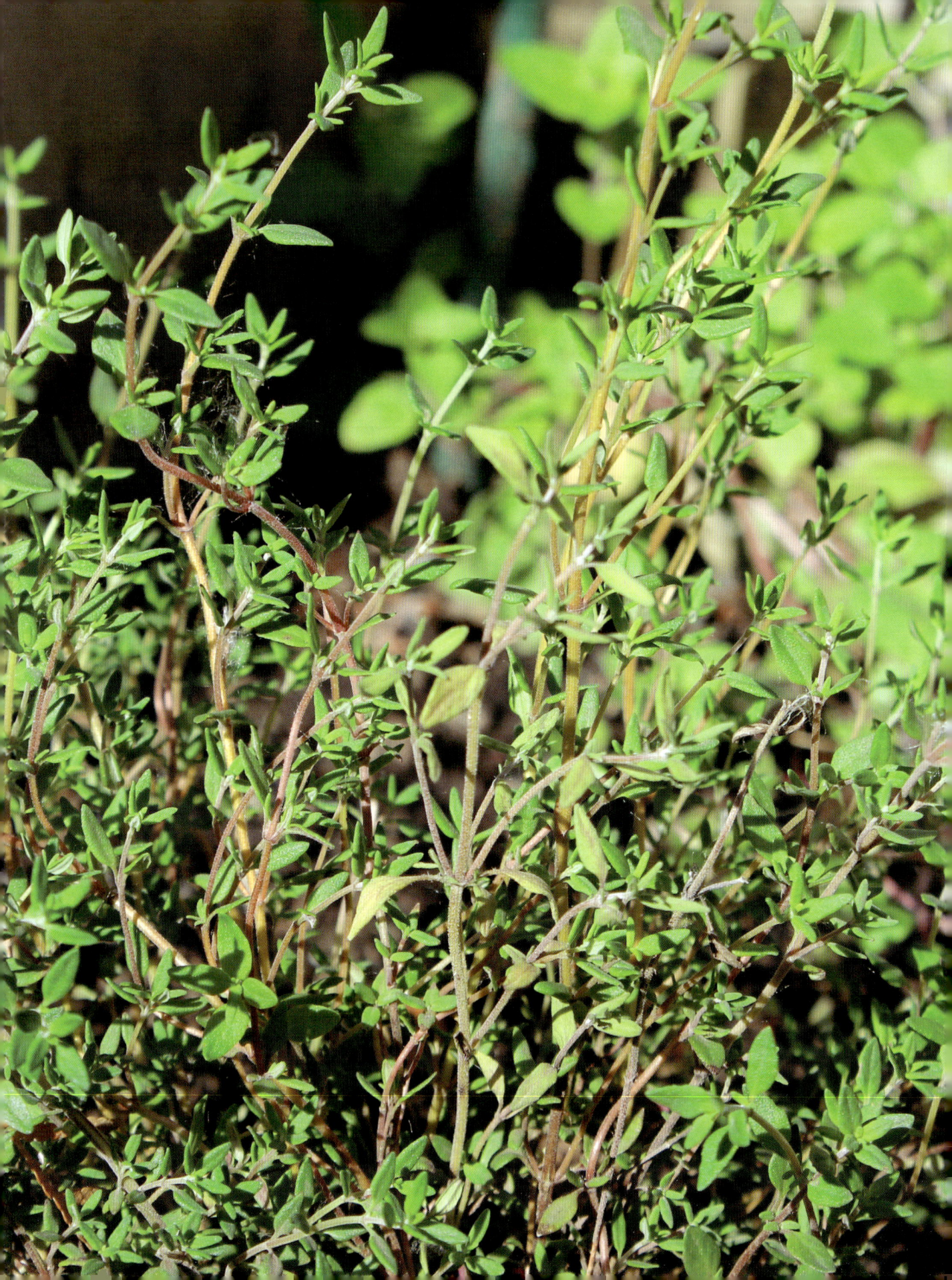

Additional Resources & Practitioners

Living a life of wellness should be a long, but lovely, journey. Following the completion of my Nutritional Therapy Certification, I have continued to study and learn from other clean-living, nutrition-focused organizations and practitioners. I can very confidently recommend each of the websites listed below as a reputable, continuing education resource to accompany you on your own path to find wellness. Never stop learning, and always enjoy the journey.

Environmental Working Group
www.ewg.org

Michael Greger, MD
www.Nutritionfacts.org

Suzy Cohen, RPH
www.suzycohen.com

Mark Hyman, MD
www.drhyman.com

Josh Axe, DNM, DC, CNS
www.draxe.com

Joseph Mercola, DO
www.mercola.com

Drew Ramsey, MD
www.drewramseymd.com

And for your viewing pleasure, check out *GMO OMG*, a 2013 documentary available on YouTube, Netflix, Amazon Prime Video, Google Play movies, or FREE from your public library.

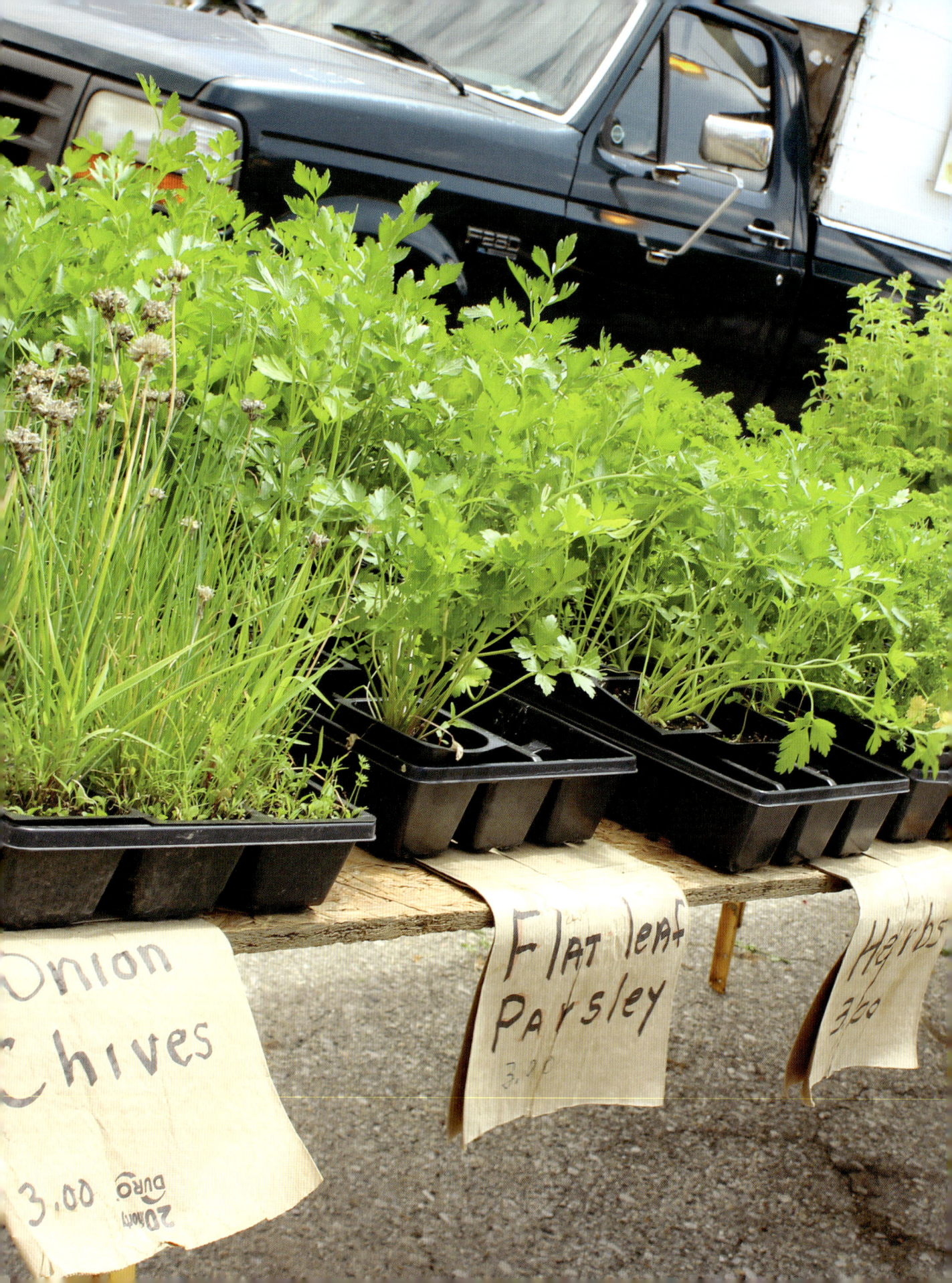

Index By Ingredient

A

almond butter 61, 77, 95, 115, 127, 135, 139, 141, 143, 145, 149, 151, 155

almonds 17, 27, 29, 41, 117, 133

apples 31, 79

artichoke 97, 115, 117

arugula 25, 69, 117, 123

asparagus 41, 49, 117

avocado 17, 25, 27, 37, 47, 51, 69, 71, 83, 93, 99, 107, 111, 123

B

bananas 139, 145, 151, 153

beans 35, 37, 51, 53, 55, 57, 99, 107, 117, 125, 147

beef 67, 71, 73, 77, 83
    chuck roast 67
    flank steak 77
    shoulder roast 67

beets 103

bell pepper 23, 25, 27, 33, 35, 49, 51, 53, 57, 61, 63, 69, 71, 77, 83, 101, 107, 115

black beans 107, 147

bok choy 77

broccoli 45, 55, 77

C

cabbage 29, 31

cacao nibs 147, 149, 153

cacao powder 147, 151, 153

capers 97, 105

carrot 29, 33, 45, 47, 63, 73, 89, 91, 115, 119, 145

cashews 17, 59, 91, 113, 115, 123, 133

cauliflower 29, 39, 103, 117

cherries 31, 35, 85, 117, 149

chia seeds 133, 139

chicken 27, 85

chickpeas 23, 61, 125

coconut 17, 31, 41, 67, 69, 71, 73, 77, 83, 85, 133, 135, 137, 139, 141, 143, 145, 149, 153, 155, 157
    coconut cream 141, 153
    coconut milk 77
    coconut water 137, 157
    flaked coconut 133
    shredded coconut 133

coconut milk 61, 127

crab 69

cranberries 71, 79

cucumber 23, 25, 35, 39, 73, 101, 129, 137

curry paste 77, 127

D

dandelion greens 89

dates 133, 143, 151, 157

E

eggplant 61, 93

G

ginger 29, 59, 61, 85, 135, 149

grape leaves 125

green chilis 51, 61, 83, 107

green peas 23, 41, 49

H

hemp seed 69, 111, 149

honey 17, 29, 123, 137

J

jalapeño 101, 107, 111

K

kale 39, 53, 89

L

lamb 73, 121, 125

lentils 47

liquid aminos 29, 127

M

macadamia nuts 157

mango 101

maple syrup 17, 33, 135, 139, 141, 145, 147, 149, 155

mushrooms 27, 35, 57, 67, 71, 93, 113

N

non-dairy milk 115, 119, 137, 151

nutritional yeast 55, 57, 69, 71, 73, 89, 91, 105, 113, 115, 119, 121

O

oats 71, 121, 139, 147, 149, 155

olives 35, 97, 105, 117, 125

orange roughy filets 81

oranges 29, 135

P

peas 23, 41, 49

pecans 17, 33, 97, 133, 143, 149

potatoes 47, 53, 67, 79, 83, 123

pumpkin 141, 145, 155

Q

quinoa 73, 79, 119

R

radish 25, 45, 73, 83

rice 29, 41, 45, 79, 85, 119, 125

S

salmon 75, 117

sesame seeds 29, 77

shoulder roast 67

spinach 115, 117, 119, 137

sun-dried tomatoes 113, 125

sweet potato 33, 83, 123, 133

T

tahini 91, 93, 99

tamari 17, 29, 127

tomatoes 23, 35, 47, 63, 73, 81, 85, 103, 105, 113, 117, 125, 129

tomato paste 83

tuna 41, 129

turkey 71, 79, 83

W

walnuts 17, 89, 93, 117, 119, 125, 133, 143, 145, 149

Y

yellow squash 27

Z

zucchini 27, 103

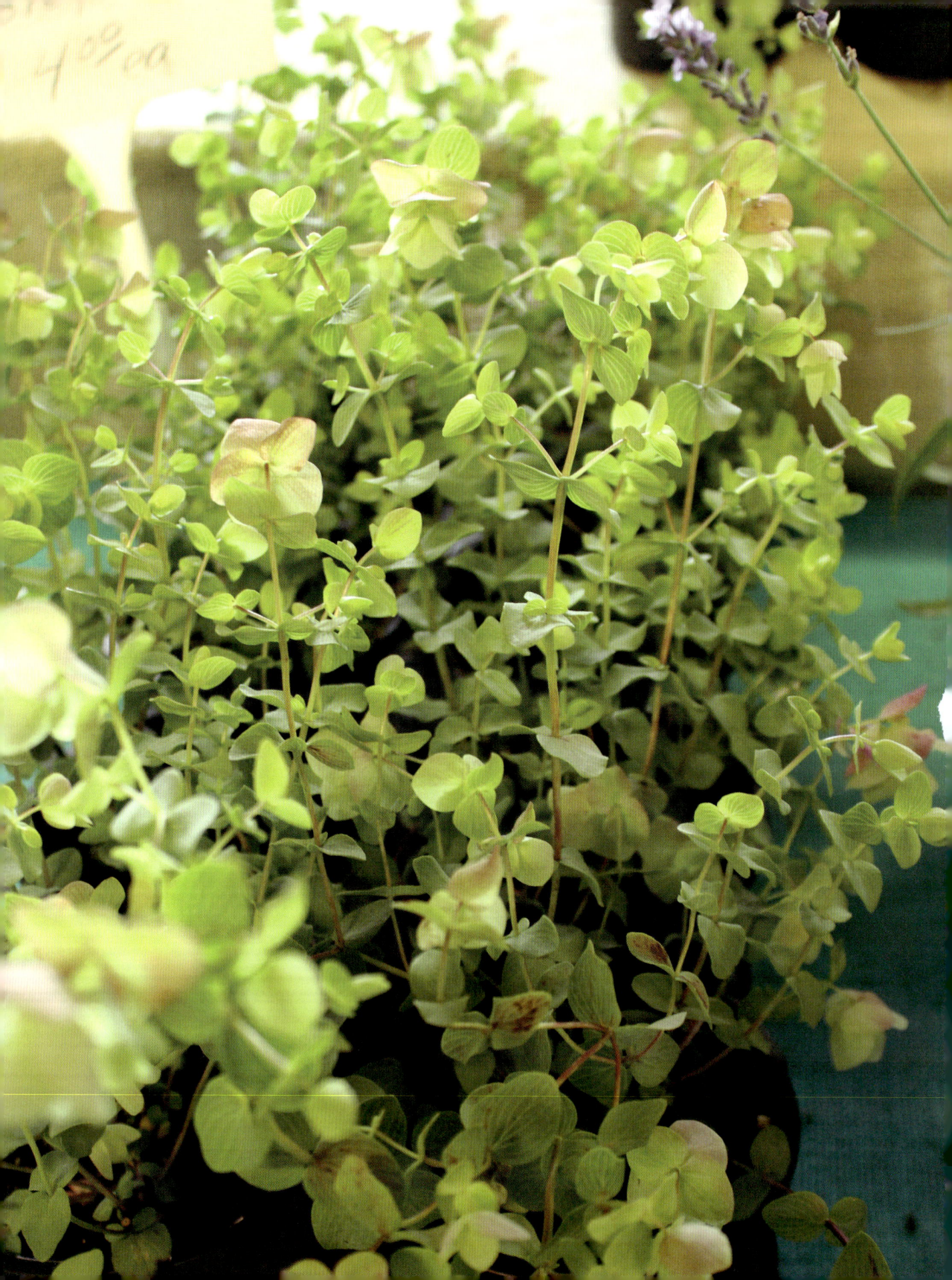

Index by Recipe Title

A
Accent Inspiring Puttanesca 105
Addressing the Dressing 95
Autumn Inspired Biscuits 155

B
Bangin' Black Bean Dip 107
Beauteous Butternut Squash Lasagna 119
Black Beans in Brownies? 147

C
Carrot Cake Inspired Banana Bread 145
Chicken Satay for your Partay 127
Cleansing Radish Ceviche 25
Cleverly Sweetened Cabbage Soup 63
Comforting Curry Stew 61
Creamy Asparagus Bisque 49
Curried Beef Stir Fry 77

D
Date Filled Delights 143
Date Night Sweet Potatoes 123
Delicious Daily Smoothie 137

E
Easy Energy Bites 133
Ella's Favorite Mango Salsa 101

F
For the Love of Cumin Chicken Chili 51
Fun Times Mocha Ice Dream 153

G
Gorgeous Ginger, Cashew Carrot Soup 59
Grateful for Green Beans 37

H
Hearty Lentil Stew 47
Herb Spring Salad with Jasmine Rice 41

I
"I'll Bring the Salad" Salad 35

K
Kicked up Chicken Salad in Lettuce Cups 111

L
Let Them Eat Artichoke Dip 115
Lovely Lemon Chia Seed Muffins 139

M
Mighty Mushroom Bisque 57

N
No Reason to be Crabby with these Crab Cakes 69
Not my Grandma's Grape Leaves 125
Not Quite Noah's Stuffed Mushrooms 113

O
Olive a Good Tapenade 97
Orange & Spice & Everything Nice Cookies 135

P
Party Worthy Pumpkin Mousse 141
Pesto Please! 89
Please Eat Pot Roast 67
Please Pass the Meatballs 121
Pleasing Pea Salad 23

R
Roasted Eggplant & Wild Mushroom Dip 93
Roasted Veggie Salad with Warm Maple Pecan Vinaigrette 33

S
Savor your Sunday with Braised Cabbage with Apples 31
Simple Citrus Cajun Salmon 75
Slow Cooked, Sweetly Spiced Chicken 85
Smoky Sweet Potato Chowder 43
Snack on this! Roasted Carrot and White Bean Hummus 99
Spreadable Cashew Cheese 91
Summertime Stuffed Peppers 73
Supremely Delicious Broccoli Soup 55
Sweet Po-Tacos 83

T
Take Me to Hawaii Please, Pudding 157
Taste of the Town 117
Taste of Venice Orange Roughy 81
Thanksgiving on a Tuesday 79
Too Easy Tuna and Tomato Boats 129
Traditional Tabbouleh with a Twist 39
Truly Tasty Turkey Meatloaf 71

V
Vacation at Home Asian Slaw 29
Valentine Marinara 103
Val's Decadent Chocolate Mousse 151
Veggie Skewers on the Barbie 27

W
Waste not, Want not Vegetable Broth 45
Wonderfully Warming Chocolate Cherry Crumble 149

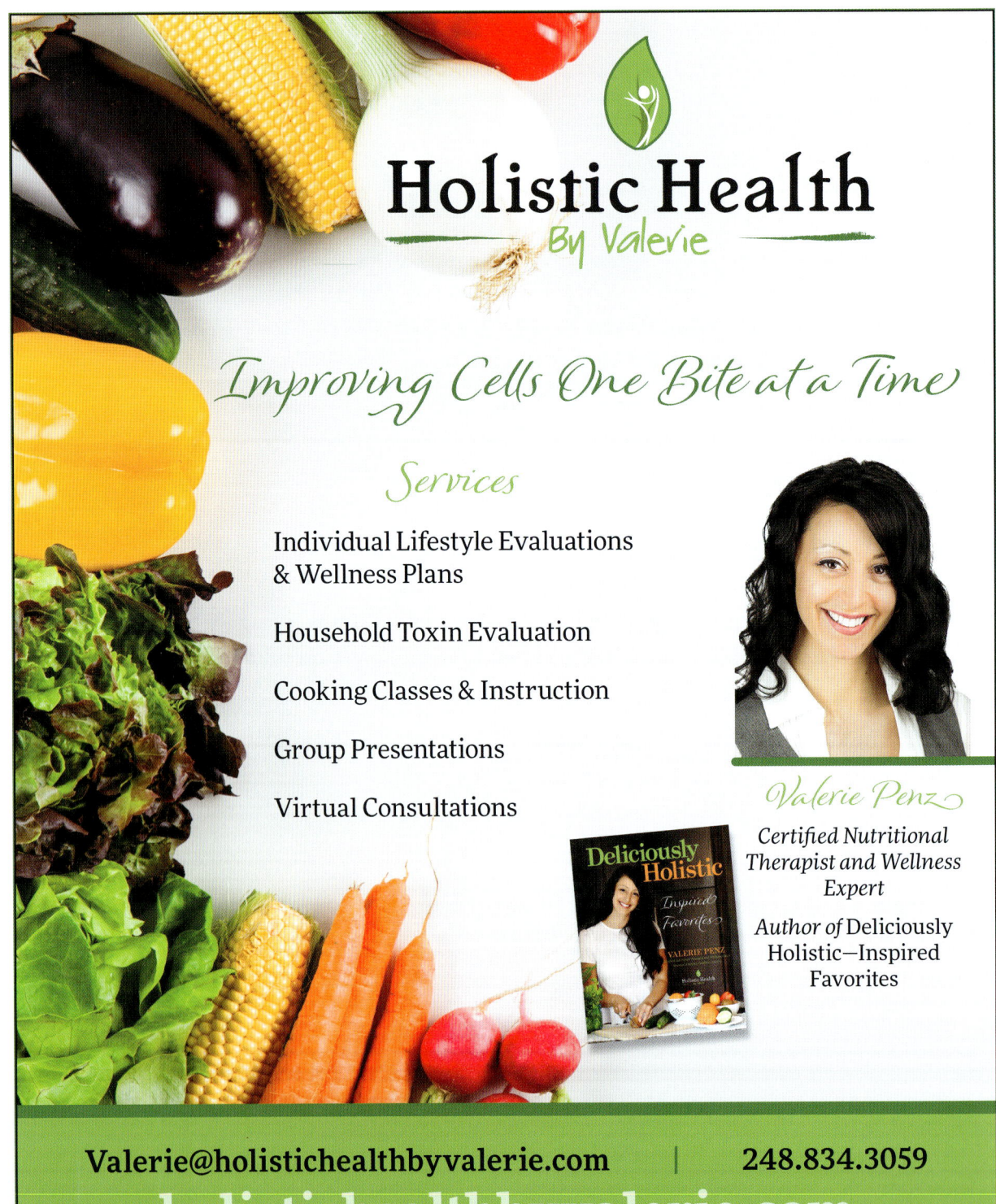